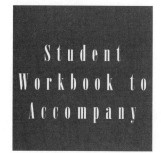

Student Workbook to Accompany

Microbiology
Principles and Health
Science Applications

D1073228

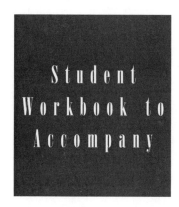

Microbiology
Principles and Health
Science Applications

Student Workbook to Accompany

Lois M. Bergquist, PhD
Professor of Microbiology
Los Angeles Valley College
Van Nuys, California

Barbara Pogosian, MS
Professor, Biology Department
Golden West College
Huntington Beach, California

W.B. Saunders Company
A Harcourt Health Sciences Company
Philadelphia London New York St. Louis Sydney Toronto

W.B. Saunders Company

A Harcourt Health Sciences Company

The Curtis Center
Independence Square West
Philadelphia, Pennsylvania 19106-3399

Student Workbook to Accompany   ISBN 0-7216-7664-2
Microbiology Principles and Health Science Applications

Printed in the United States of America.

Last digit is the print number: 9 8 7 6 5 4 3 2 1

Acknowledgements

Writing a study guide to accompany a textbook is like trying to place ourselves in the roles of both student and teacher. We have been working as teachers for many years, and our experience has been honed and polished by the efforts our students make to do what we ask of them. We hope they have understood that the motivation behind our actions is to increase their knowledge and skills of microbiology, which will assist them in their careers. Our education is always enhanced by the thousands of students we have worked with, and we acknowledge their invaluable contributions to our own understanding of the processes of teaching and learning. We acknowledge our teachers and the academic scholars who helped us to see what a microbiology education requires. For you, the new student, we acknowledge your willingness, by buying this book and using it, to improve your understanding of microbiology.

TABLE OF CONTENTS

UNIT 1

An Introduction to Microbiology

UNIT 2

Growth, Metabolism, and Variation

UNIT 3

Major Groups of Microorganisms

UNIT 4

UNIT 5

UNIT 6

UNIT 7

Study Tips

You are sure to complete this course successfully with a good understanding and increased knowledge and skills of microbiology with some planning. Decide what you want to achieve as a student in this course and then write your decision down as a statement of intention, so you'll remember it. Look at your written statement frequently to inspire you to continue working. Begin with a positive statement such as "I will" or "I want to have." Avoid using the word try, as in "I will try" or you won't give yourself the chance to achieve your goals. Here are some behaviors that will ensure that you accomplish your goals.

1. **Attend** class on time every class meeting.
2. **Listen** carefully and take clear notes on the lectures in each class meeting. Survey your notes after the lecture to see if you need to add something to make them clear and complete.
3. **Read** the textbook and write additional comments into your lecture notes based on your reading.
4. **Make notes** of any class assignments and their due dates. Mark these due dates on your calendar.
5. **On your calendar, mark the times you will study** or work on these assignments. Consider these times appointments with yourself; they are. Keep these appointments.
6. **Write** a statement of intention that describes what you want to get out of this class. The statement will be more helpful if you identify how this class will relate to your career choices and other courses.

   Statement of intention: _____

   _____

   _____

   _____

   _____

7. **Prepare** a study location at home where you can keep essential items, such as a type-writer or computer, dictionary, textbooks, pens, pencils, paper, stapler, music system (if you need music), exercise equipment (if you need to stretch or work out the kinks), and anything else that you will need regularly to work.
8. **Visit the library** to find out what services are provided to students. For example, computers, quiet rooms, hours of service. Use these services.
9. If you think microbiology will be difficult, **find out** if there are tutoring services at your campus. Sign up early for a tutor.
10. When you have a long assignment with many parts to it, such as writing a research paper or studying for an examination, **break the assignment down into several smaller assignments** that would take 15 to 30 minutes to complete. Work every day on another portion of the large assignment, until you are done.
11. **Begin working early** on your assignments. Don't wait until you have only one or two days left before you have to turn it in.
12. **Ask for help** every time you need it.
13. **Keep working** on the course assignments even when you are having difficulty understanding the material. Read tip #12.

Using This Study Guide to Achieve Your Goals

This study guide is a workbook for you to practice answering multiple-choice, fill-in-the-blank and matching questions. Some crossword puzzles and figures for you to label are included to assist you with the vocabulary of microbiology and its application to biological processes. Short-answer questions will help you practice writing clear, complete answers to essay questions, as well as achieve a greater level of understanding of the material.

Each chapter in the textbook is represented by a chapter in this study guide. The chapters are divided into three sections: Chapter Learning Objectives, Study Outline, and Study Questions for Chapter Objectives. Each chapter has several Learning Objectives to guide your study of the chapter's content. The Study Outline presents a brief outline of the entire chapter for your quick review before and after a lecture, and before an examination. The Study Questions give you a chance to practice using terminology in a format similar to an examination.

Chapter Learning Objectives

Read these objectives first when you begin to study a chapter. There are several learning objectives for each chapter, and several more may be added by your instructor. We know these are helpful in focusing your attention on the reading of the textbook, so that you can find answers as you read. In some courses, learning objectives are not given to students to direct their study, yet this study guide will give you a foundation for your study. These objectives form the basis for the study questions you find in this guide.

If your instructor has additional learning objectives or different learning objectives, then use the textbook, study guide, and lecture notes to help you study. The study questions will help you learn the vocabulary of microbiology, and the biological principles involved. To help yourself, you may use the study guide as a model for writing your own tests, based on the learning objectives provided by your instructor.

Study Outline

Use this outline to help you understand what your teacher will present in a lecture program. After the lecture, read the outline to help you understand your own notes. Write additional comments based on the outline and the textbook, to make your lecture notes more complete. When you are preparing for an examination, complete lecture notes will be extremely helpful.

Reading the Study Outline several days before you take an examination will remind you of the essential points in the chapter. If an item in the outline does not sound familiar, return to your notes from the lecture and the textbook, to review the material. Frequent review of your notes, the textbook, and the Study Outline will help you understand the material with less and less difficulty—and eventually with ease and confidence. Where you still have difficulty understanding the material, be sure to ask your instructor for assistance early. The instructor can provide answers that will help you break through in your understanding of the material, and will save you time.

Study Questions for Chapter Objectives

Many different types of questions are in the study guide so that you can practice taking different types of test questions. Some instructors may use objective-type questions such as matching, multiple-choice, and fill-in-the-blank exclusively. Other instructors may focus on having students write short and long essay answers. Instructors may also use a combination of objective questions and essay questions.

Answer the questions in each chapter as if you were preparing for an examination. The answer key for each chapter is printed in the back of the book. Refer to the answer key only after you have finished answering the questions. Then, after checking your answers, decide what topics you need to study in more detail. If you use the answer key too frequently, you will not adequately test your memory and understanding of the material.

By answering the questions using a soft pencil, you will be able to erase the answers and answer the questions a second or third time to improve your memory and understanding of the material. This type of studying is called a "drill" because it provides repetition.

Some students study a course by relating new material to material they have already studied and understood. Often, these students write essay questions well because they understand the steps in a process and how the steps relate to other similar processes. This study guide gives you a way to develop an understanding and mastery of the material, so that you form new relationships between what you already understand and the new material.

Essay questions often compare the similarity in items and contrast those items for their differences. For example, an essay question might ask you to compare and contrast the cellular structures of procaryote and eucaryote cell types. First, you would have to understand the two cell types; then you would have to remember the structures that are similar in both cell types, and write about their similarities. Next, you would recall where the two cell types are different and write about those differences. If you have taken other biology courses, this kind of question will be a review of some material on cell structures, which you can use to answer the question, and perhaps the procaryote cell type is the new material that you must learn and recall in order to answer the type of question mentioned above.

The best way to prepare for essay-type examinations is to write essay-type questions and answer them in writing. The short-answer essay questions in this study guide provide opportunities for you to practice answering essay questions. Plus, you can write and answer your own sample questions based on your interpretation of what your instructor thinks is important. Check the textbook to see if your answer is complete. Ask your instructor to look at your answers and to make suggestions on how to improve them.

We wish you many wonderful experiences as you increase your awareness of the microbial world and its impact on the environment, human health, food, sanitation, water quality, and many other aspects of our lives here on earth. Use the study guide to provide you with the very best opportunity to achieve your career and academic goals.

Course Assignments

Date	Assignment-Chapters, Pages	Due Date	Completed (✓)

Course Assignments

Date	Assignment-Chapters, Pages	Due Date	Completed (✓)

AN INTRODUCTION TO MICROBIOLOGY

CHAPTER 1

Discovery and Diversity of the Microbial World

Learning Objectives

1. Explain the methods used to disprove the theory of spontaneous generation.
2. Describe the origin of the germ theory of disease.
3. Name the contributions of the early pioneers in microbiology.
4. Explain the basis of vaccination in prevention of infectious diseases.
5. Name the two patterns of cellular organization found in microorganisms.
6. Explain why acellular particles cannot be classified as procaryotes or eucaryotes.

Study Outline

The Origin of Life

1. The belief in the spontaneous generation of life from nonliving matter was introduced by Aristotle more than 2,000 years ago.
2. A recipe for spontaneously generating mice from rags and grains was proposed by van Helmont.

The Controversy Over Spontaneous Generation

1. Francesco Redi temporarily resolved the questions on the origin of life with an experiment showing that decaying meat did not spontaneously generate flies.
2. Antony van Leeuwenhoek was the first to record observations on microorganisms.

3. Conflicting results on the origin of microorganisms in heated broths were obtained by John Needham and Lazzaro Spallanzani.

4. Louis Pasteur disproved the theory of spontaneous generation by heating broths in swan-necked flasks.

5. John Tyndall and Ferdinand Cohn described heat-stable and heat-resistant forms of microbial life.

The Germ Theory of Disease

1. Frascatorius proposed that living organisms caused disease.

2. Oliver Wendell Holmes and Ignaz Semmelweis reduced the number of infections in maternity wards by teaching handwashing techniques to medical staff.

3. Louis Pasteur discovered the role of microorganisms in alcoholic fermentation and wine spoilage.

4. The number of undesirable microorganisms is reduced by a heating process developed by Louis Pasteur; this process is now called pasteurization.

5. Pasteur discovered the bacterium that causes puerperal fever in the blood of infected patients.

6. Joseph Lister reduced the risk of postsurgical infections by using carbolic acid as a surgical aerosol, and in dressings.

The Developing Science of Microbiology: Koch's Techniques

1. Robert Koch is credited with pure culture techniques for the growth of microorganisms, and techniques for staining microorganisms for microscopic examination.

2. Koch established guidelines known as "Koch's postulates," used for obtaining proof of the cause of an infectious disease.

3. Koch's postulates cannot be fulfilled if a disease occurs only in humans or if the disease agent will not grow on artificial culture media.

The Beginnings of Immunology

1. Edward Jenner is credited with injecting cowpox material into skin as a protection against smallpox; this process is called vaccination.

2. Pasteur developed vaccines for chicken cholera, anthrax, and rabies by a process of attenuation.

3. Elie Metchnikoff formulated the theory of phagocytosis to explain resistance to infectious disease.

4. Paul Ehrlich proposed that components of the blood were responsible for immunity.

The Discovery of Antimicrobial Agents

1. Paul Ehrlich earned the title "Father of Chemotherapy" when he introduced Salvarsan for the treatment of syphilis.

2. Gerhard Domagk showed that sulfa drugs were effective treatments against many bacterial infections.

3. Alexander Fleming's discovery of penicillin from the mold *Penicillium notatum* expanded research efforts for other antimicrobial agents.

Microorganisms: The Natural Jewelry of the Earth

1. Microorganisms can be unicellular or multicellular, or can lack cellular organization.

2. The metric units used for measuring microorganisms are micrometers (μm) and nanometers (nm).

Classification and Nomenclature of Microorganisms

1. The three-kingdom classification system proposed by Ernst Haeckel in 1866 placed microorganisms in a separate kingdom, Protista.

2. Carl Woese described three domains of organisms in the 1970s, dividing them into Bacteria, Archaea, and Eucarya.

3. The six-kingdom classification system places cellular organisms into the kingdoms Archaea, Eubacteria, Protista, Fungi, Plantae, and Animalia.

4. Bergey's Manual classifies Eubacteria and Archaea in one kingdom called Procaryotae.

5. Carolus Linnaeus introduced a binomial system of nomenclature that uses genus and species names.

6. The genus name is capitalized, and the species name is spelled in lowercase letters.

7. The binomial name is printed in italicized letters when appearing in a publication (as in *Escherichia coli*) and underlined when handwritten (as in <u>Escherichia</u> <u>coli</u>).

The Major Groups of Microorganisms

1. The major groups of cellular microorganisms are: bacteria (including archaea), algae, protozoa, and fungi.

2. The presence of membrane-bound organelles is one factor of cellular organization that places the algae, fungi, and protozoa into the eucaryotic group of microorganisms.

3. The bacteria and archaea do not have membrane-bound organelles, and they are the only members of the procaryotic group.

4. The acellular viruses depend on host cells for their existence.

Archaea

1. Archaebacteria survive in the absence of oxygen, in nutrient-barren environments, and in extremes of temperature or salinity.

2. These forms of life differ from other procaryotes and the eucaryotes in chemical and structural characteristics.

Bacteria

1. All eubacteria, except rickettsias and chlamydias, can live independently of host cells.

2. A majority of bacteria produce materials that sustain other forms of life.

3. Some eubacteria cause life-threatening diseases that affect world population and the quality of life.

Microbial Eucarya

1. Some molecules of eucarya resemble those in archaea more than bacteria.

2. Microbial eucarya are algae, protozoa, and fungi.

Acellular Particles

1. Viruses depend on bacterial, archaeal, or eukaryotic host cells for their replication; viruses are parasites of cells.

2. Most viruses are visible only with an electron microscope.

 Study Questions for Chapter Objectives

Match the names with a letter for the experimental method from choices in column A, and with the letter for the conclusion of the experiment from choices in column B. Write the letters in the space for each column. Some choices may be used more than once.

Column A   **Column B**

————————   ————————

————————   ————————

————————   ————————

————————   ————————

————————   ————————

————————   ————————

1. Francesco Redi

2. Lazzaro Spallanzani

3. John Needham

4. Louis Pasteur

5. John Tyndall

6. Ferdinand Cohn

Column A: Methods

a. Sterile, swan-necked flasks of broth
b. Prolonged heating of heat-stable and heat-sensitive
c. Boiled mutton broth in corked flasks
d. Decaying meat in open jar and decaying meat in gauze-covered jar
e. Boiled mutton broth in airtight flask

Column B: Conclusions

A. Intermittent heating killed cells that germinated from endospores.
B. Even with air exposure, the sterilized broth did not spontaneously generate cells.
C. Microbial growth occurred in a few days, spontaneously.
D. Microbial growth did not occur spontaneously in an airtight flask.
E. Maggots on meat arose from eggs laid there by flies, not by spontaneous generation.
F. Called heat-stable forms of bacteria, endospores.

7. In a short essay or outline, describe the germ theory of disease and the contributions of the following people: Frascatorius, Semmelweis, Chamberland, Pasteur, Holmes, Joubert, and Lister.

_____

_____

_____

_____

_____

_____

_____

Match the name of a microbiologist in column B with a contribution in column A. A name from column B may be used more than once.

Column A

_____ 8. Introduced smallpox vaccination
_____ 9. Recommended agar to solidify media
_____ 10. Described phagocytosis
_____ 11. Developed chicken cholera vaccine
_____ 12. Used carbolic acid in surgery
_____ 13. Developed pure culture techniques to grow bacteria in the laboratory
_____ 14. Made first simple lens microscope and could see bacteria
_____ 15. Developed postulates to demonstrate that a microorganism caused disease
_____ 16. Recorded first descriptions of microorganisms
_____ 17. Observed membrane-bound organelles
_____ 18. Developed heating process to reduce numbers of bacteria and kill pathogens
_____ 19. Disproved spontaneous generation
_____ 20. Developed Salvarsan
_____ 21. Recommended handwashing between patients to reduce infections and death after childbirth
_____ 22. Discovered penicillin
_____ 23. Developed vaccine for rabies
_____ 24. Developed two-part dish for cultivating microorganisms
_____ 25. Solved problem of infections in wine in France

Column B

a. van Leeuwenhoek
b. Pasteur
c. Metchnikoff
d. Koch
e. Fleming
f. Ehrlich
g. Jenner
h. Lister
i. Semmelweis
j. Chatton
k. Petri
l. Hesse
m. Chamberland

Match the contribution of the following persons or methods in the development of vaccinations.

_____ 26. Lady Montague
_____ 27. Pasteur
_____ 28. Jenner
_____ 29. Chamberland
_____ 30. Chinese technique

a. Cholera bacteria weakened by a long period of broth cultivation induced immunity after injection into chickens
b. Material from smallpox scabs placed in a vein gave lifelong immunity
c. Vaccines to rabies, anthrax, and chicken cholera were developed
d. Dried smallpox crusts placed in the nose
e. Material from cowpox lesions introduced into the skin by punctures

Match the pattern of cellular organization to its name.

_____ 31. No organelles
_____ 32. Membrane-bound organelles
_____ 33. Membrane-bound nucleus
_____ 34. Nuclear material is free in cytoplasm
_____ 35. Many internal membranes

a. Procaryote
b. Eucaryote

Match the microorganism in column A with the pattern of cellular organization from column B.

Column A

_____ 36. Bacteria
_____ 37. Viruses
_____ 38. Algae
_____ 39. Fungi
_____ 40. Protozoa

Column B

a. Procaryotic
b. Eucaryotic
c. Neither *a* nor *b* choices

41. Explain why acellular particles cannot be classified as procaryotes or eucaryotes. Identify what an acellular particle is.

_____

_____

_____

_____

_____

42. Why did it take so long to disprove the theory of spontaneous generation?

_____

_____

_____

_____

_____

_____

43. Explain why Semmelweis's recommendations on handwashing are not limited to maternity wards.

_____

_____

_____

_____

_____

44. How do phagocytic cells defend us against microbial invaders?

_____

_____

_____

45. Why are classification schemes for microorganisms useful?

_____

_____

_____

_____

CHAPTER 2
The Chemistry of Life

Learning Objectives

1. Name the four major elements found in cells.
2. Define element, atom, compound, molecule, and mixture.
3. Explain how electrons in the outer shell determine the behavior of atoms.
4. Describe three types of chemical bonds.
5. Explain the origin of chemical symbols.
6. Describe two major types of chemical reactions.
7. Name the four major organic molecules found in living things and the elements they contain.

Study Outline

Elements and Compounds
1. All cells contain the elements carbon, hydrogen, oxygen, and nitrogen.
2. The atom is the smallest portion of an element that enters into a chemical reaction.
3. A molecule has two or more atoms.
4. A mixture contains two or more elements or compounds that have not reacted together.

Chemical Shorthand
1. Elements are represented by abbreviations known as symbols.
2. A symbol may consist of a single capitalized letter or the first two letters of its name.
3. Compounds are represented by abbreviations called formulas.
4. Subscripts are used to express numbers of atoms of an element, in a molecule of a compound.

Functional Groups
1. Certain atoms consistently associate with other atoms to form functional groups, such as an amino group (NH_2).

2. Functional groups behave differently than the individual atoms of which they are composed, and have their own valences.

The Structure of Atoms
1. Atoms contain three major types of particles: protons, neutrons, and electrons.
2. The atomic nucleus contains positively charged (+) protons and uncharged neutrons.
3. The negatively charged (−) electrons move around the nucleus in pathways called shells.
4. Electrons in the outermost shell determine the behavior of an atom.
5. The number of electrons equals the number of protons.
6. The atomic number equals the number of protons in an atom; the atomic weight equals the sum of protons and neutrons of an atom.

Energy Relationships of Atoms

1. The loss, gain, or sharing of electrons produces an energy relationship between atoms called a chemical bond.

2. An atom can form bonds for every unpaired electron in the outermost orbit.

3. Bonds are classified as ionic, covalent, or hydrogen.

Ionic Bonds

1. Ionic bonds are formed when electrons are transferred from the outer shell of one atom to the outer shell of another atom.

2. The loss of electrons causes an atom to have a positive charge; the gain of electrons causes an atom to have a negative charge.

Covalent Bonds

1. Covalent bonds are formed when electrons of atoms are shared.

2. If an atom of carbon forms bonds with less than four atoms of hydrogen, then double or triple covalent bonds are formed.

3. The term "unsaturated" describes compounds that contain double or triple covalent bonds.

4. A pull of the same magnitude on shared electrons creates a nonpolar covalent bond.

5. Pulls of unequal magnitude on shared electrons create a polar covalent bond.

Hydrogen Bonds

1. The unequal sharing of electrons in a molecule that contains hydrogen causes hydrogen to bond with atoms of electronegative elements.

2. Hydrogen bonds are formed by water molecules when electronegative oxygen attracts an atom of hydrogen in another water molecule.

3. Large numbers of hydrogen bonds stabilize molecules of proteins and nucleic acids.

Energy Content of Bonds

1. The energy of bonds is measured in kilocalories per mole.

2. Covalent bonds contain 80 to 110 kilocalories per mole; hydrogen bonds yield 4 to 6 kilocalories per mole.

3. Ionic bonds store approximately 5 kilocalories per mole.

Types of Chemical Reactions

1. Energy is required to form a chemical bond; energy is released when chemical bonds are broken.

2. Reactions may be classified as energy-requiring (endergonic) or energy-liberating (exergonic).

Reversibility of Reactions

1. In theory, all chemical reactions are reversible.

2. A reaction may not be reversible if molecules are stable and environmental conditions are unchanged.

A Chemical Accounting System

1. Chemical reactions are expressed in equations that use formulas for reactants.

2. The number and types of atoms on one side of the equation must balance the number and types of atoms on the other side of the equation.

Acids, Bases, and Salts

1. The atoms of some molecules that separate (dissociate) when dissolved in water, and release hydrogen ions (H^+), are called acids.

2. Molecules that dissociate and release hydroxyl ions (OH^-) are called bases.

Measurement of Acidity (pH)

1. The acidity, or pH, of a solution is measured on a scale of 0 to 14, with the number 7 representing neutrality.

2. Solutions with a pH below 7 are acidic; solutions with a pH above 7 on the scale are alkaline.

3. A change in one unit on the scale represents a tenfold change in hydrogen ion (H^+) concentration.

The Role of Buffers

1. Chemicals known as buffers can combine with or release hydrogen ions (H^+) or hydroxyl ions (OH^-).

2. Nontoxic buffers may be added to culture media to counteract acid or alkaline waste products from cellular activity.

Organic Molecules

1. The major organic molecules associated with living things are carbohydrates, proteins, lipids, and nucleic acids.

2. Most of the carbon atoms of organic molecules are bonded to hydrogen atoms.

Carbohydrates: The Energy-Rich Molecules

1. Carbohydrates are major energy sources for all living things.
2. The empirical formula for a carbohydrate is $(CH_2O)n$, where n is equal to the number of carbon atoms in a molecule; in glucose and fructose, n is 6; in ribose, n is 5.

Monosaccharides

1. Simple carbohydrates that contain three to seven carbon (C) atoms are called monosaccharides.
2. The pentoses (five-carbon compounds) and hexoses (six-carbon compounds) occur in ring forms.

Disaccharides

1. A disaccharide is formed when two monosaccharides combine.
2. The bond formed between the two simple sugars is known as a glycosidic bond.

Polysaccharides

1. The polysaccharides contain multiple hexoses, or pentoses with numerous glycosidic bonds.
2. Cellulose is the most abundant polysaccharide in nature.

Proteins: The Determinants of Diversity

1. Proteins consist of long chains of amino acids and make up about 50 percent of all living things.
2. Enzymes that catalyze chemical reactions are proteins.
3. Amino acids contain at least one amino group (NH_2), and at least one carboxyl group (COOH).

Primary Structure

1. A peptide bond forms between two amino acids when a carboxyl group (COOH) reacts with an amino group (NH_2) and a molecule of water is lost. A long chain of amino acids is linked by peptide bonds.
2. A polypeptide contains 10 or more amino acids.
3. There are 20 commonly-occurring amino acids in nature.

Secondary Structure

1. Long chains of amino acids form helices, or pleated sheet arrangements, which are connected by hydrogen bonds.
2. A single hydrogen bond is weak, but a large number of them together account for the structural integrity of proteins.

Tertiary Structure

1. Additional coiling and folding of chains of amino acids cause proteins to become globular in shape.
2. The tertiary structure is stabilized by additional hydrogen, ionic, and disulfide bonds.
3. Hydrophobic polar side chains on an amino acid are hidden within the protein, and hydrophilic side chains are exposed.

Quaternary Structure

1. Proteins that contain more than one polypeptide chain demonstrate a quaternary structure.
2. Hydrogen bonds, ionic bonds, and hydrophobic side chains contribute to the association of peptide chains.

Conjugated Proteins

1. Proteins combine with nonprotein organic compounds or inorganic compounds to form conjugated proteins.
2. Examples of conjugated proteins are glycoproteins, lipoproteins, and nucleoproteins.

Denaturation of Proteins

1. Proteins are denatured when chemical bonds of the molecule are broken.
2. Denatured proteins are no longer biologically active.

Lipids: The Distant Cousins

1. Lipids are sparingly soluble in water, but readily soluble in organic solvents.
2. Lipids are major constituents of plasma membranes.

Simple Lipids

1. Simple lipids contain fatty acids and an alcohol.
2. Saturated fatty acids contain the maximum number of hydrogen atoms at carbon-binding sites; unsaturated fatty acids contain double bonds with less than the maximum number of hydrogen atoms at carbon-binding sites.
3. An ester bond is formed between fatty acids and glycerol, with the loss of a molecule of water.

Compound Lipids

1. Phospholipids, glycolipids, and steroids are important compound lipids.
2. The most important steroid is cholesterol.

Nucleic Acids: The Informational Molecules

1. All cellular organisms contain DNA and RNA; the viruses contain either DNA or RNA.
2. DNA stores all the cellular information and its inherited properties, especially for making RNA and proteins.
3. RNA makes proteins as specified by a base sequence on DNA.

Nucleosides and Nucleotides

1. The nitrogen bases of nucleic acids are the pyrimidines cytosine (C), thymine (T), and uracil (U), and the purines adenine (A) and cytosine (C).
2. A nucleoside consists of a pyrimidine or purine linked to a five-carbon sugar.
3. The addition of a phosphate group (PO_4) to a nucleoside forms a nucleotide–the building block of nucleic acids.

4. Nucleic acids consist of long chains of nucleotides occurring in single or double strands.

Deoxyribonucleic Acid

1. The two strands of DNA are held together by hydrogen bonds between a purine on one strand and a pyrimidine on the opposite strand; the nucleotides contain deoxyribose sugar.
2. Adenine (A) always forms hydrogen bonds with thymine (T), and cytosine (C) always forms hydrogen bonds with guanine (G) in DNA; A and T are base pairs; C and G are base pairs.
3. The pairing of nitrogen bases is known as complementarity.

Ribonucleic Acid

1. RNA has nucleotides with one of four bases: adenine, guanine, cytosine, uracil (no thymine), and the sugar ribose.
2. Messenger RNA (mRNA) and ribosomal RNA (rRNA) are single-stranded; a part of transfer RNA (tRNA) folds back on itself and appears to be double-stranded.
3. Triplets of nitrogen bases on mRNA are called codons; their complementary bases on tRNA are called anticodons.

 Study Questions for Chapter Objectives

Write the name of the chemical element represented by the following symbols, and the atomic number for each element:

1. C _____

2. N _____

3. O _____

4. H _____

Write the Latin name for the following chemical symbols, and the common name for the element:

Latin Name	Common Name
5. Cu _____	_____
6. Na _____	_____

Write the chemical symbol for the following elements:

7. Potassium _____

8. Calcium _____

9. Iodine _____

10. Sulfur _____

11. Phosphorus _____

12. Chlorine _____

13. Iron _____

14. Magnesium _____

Identify the two names in items 7 to 14 with chemical symbols that have an origin in a Latin name.

15. _____ _____

(Can you identify the Latin name?)

16. _____ _____

(Can you identify the Latin name?)

17. For the other names in items 7 to 14, the chemical symbols are derived from what property of the name?

_____

_____

_____

_____

_____

Define the following terms by identifying the chemical that matches it. Some terms can be matched by more than one lettered choice.

Key for 18-22:

_____ 18. Element
_____ 19. Atom
_____ 20. Compound
_____ 21. Molecule
_____ 22. Mixture

a. Carbon dioxide (CO_2)
b. Nitrogen gas (N_2)
c. Air, N_2, O_2, plus other material
d. One unit of H_2O
e. Hydrogen (H)

Write a check mark in the appropriate column for the type of chemical bond in each molecule in the table.

Name of Molecule	Type of Chemical Bond		
	Ionic	Covalent	Hydrogen
23. NaCl			
24. H_2			
25. C_2H_4			
26. C_2H_2			
27. H_2O to H_2O			
28. Ribose			
29. Peptide bond			
30. Protein secondary structure			
31. Protein tertiary structure			
32. Stearic acid			
33. $C_6H_{12}O_6$ (glucose)			
34. $AgNO_3$			
35. NaOH			

____ 36. Identify which pair shows a correct relationship:
   a. Peptide bond: carboxyl group bound to amino group
   b. Peptide bond: glycine-alanine
   c. Peptide bond: protein
   d. None of *a* through *c* choices
   e. All of *a* through *c* choices

____ 37. Identify the appropriate pair:
   a. Glycosidic bond: peptide
   b. Glycosidic bond: glucose-glucose
   c. Glycosidic bond: stearic acid
   d. None of *a* through *c* choices
   e. All of *a* through *c* choices

____ 38. Identify the appropriate pair:
   a. Disulfide bond: starch
   b. Disulfide bond: protein
   c. Disulfide bond: lipids
   d. None of *a* through *c* choices
   e. All of *a* through *c* choices

____ 39. Identify the appropriate pair:
   a. Ester bond: protein
   b. Ester bond: peptide
   c. Ester bond: glycerol-fatty acid
   d. None of *a* through *c* choices
   e. All of *a* through *c* choices

____ 40. Fatty acids with one bond between the carbon atoms are:
   a. Bonded
   b. Saturated
   c. Unsaturated
   d. Denatured
   e. Neutral

____ 41. Fatty acids with two or three bonds between some carbon atoms are:
   a. Bonded
   b. Saturated
   c. Unsaturated
   d. Denatured
   e. Neutral

____ 42. When electrons are transferred from one atom to another, the bond is:

____ 43. When electrons are shared between atoms, the bond is:

____ 44. When polar covalent molecules attract other polar covalent molecules between H^+ and negatively charged atoms, the bond is:

Key for 42-44:
   a. Hydrogen
   b. Covalent
   c. Ionic
   d. None of *a* through *c* choices
   e. All of *a* through *c* choices

____ 45. A reaction that requires energy in order to proceed is called:

____ 46. A reaction that releases energy as it proceeds is called:

Key for 45-46:
   a. Valence
   b. Exergonic
   c. Reversible
   d. Endergonic
   e. Ionic

47. Why is it necessary to know valences to write formulas correctly?

_____

_____

_____

_____

_____

_____

48. Explain how electrons in the outer shell determine the behavior of atoms in forming bonds. Be sure to state the octet principle, and explain the concept of valence.

_____

_____

_____

_____

_____

_____

_____

49. Name four major organic molecules found in living organisms and the elements contained within them.

_____

_____

_____

50. Write the definition of pH and explain why buffers are added to microbiological culture media.

_____

_____

_____

_____

51. If a segment of DNA contains the following triplets of bases, construct the mRNA with its appropriate codons, and the complementary strand of tRNA with its appropriate anticodons.

     TAC CAT TAG GAG CCC ATT

     mRNA: ____ ____ ____ ____ ____ ____

     tRNA: ____ ____ ____ ____ ____ ____

52. What is meant by the polarity of a molecule?

     _____

     _____

     _____

     _____

53. If rain has a pH of less than 5.6, it is called acid rain. Major compounds responsible for acidity of the rain are sulfur dioxide (SO_2) and nitrogen dioxide (NO_2). What are the sources of the dioxides? How does acid rain affect aquatic life? Why would lakes that contain basins of carbonate rock be less affected by acid rain?

     _____

     _____

     _____

     _____

CHAPTER 3

Observation of Microorganisms

Learning Objectives

1. Describe seven types of microscopes and one specific use for each of them.
2. Differentiate between the magnifying and resolving power of a microscope.
3. Explain how the magnification of the light microscope is determined.
4. Compare the image obtained with a transmission electron microscope to that obtained with a scanning electron microscope.
5. Explain the need for a variety of staining techniques.

Study Outline

Types of Microscopes

1. Most microorganisms can be seen with a light microscope.
2. Detailed studies of cellular structures and viruses require the better resolution and greater magnification of an electron microscope.

The Bright-Field Microscope

1. The bright-field microscope is a compound-lens microscope because it uses two sets of lenses. The magnified image from an objective lens is magnified again by the ocular lens.
2. The magnified size of an object is obtained by multiplying the enlarging powers of the objective and ocular lenses.
3. The resolving power of a microscope is the smallest distance that is visible between two adjacent points.

The Dark-Field Microscope

1. A dark-field microscope has one or more special condensers to adjust the path of light away from the objective lens.

2. Microorganisms bend the light into the objective lens so they are seen as light objects against a dark background.
3. The uses of dark-field microscopy include visualization of spirochetes and capsules of microorganisms.

The Phase-Contrast Microscope

1. A phase-contrast microscope has a special condenser and an objective lens assembly that accentuate differences in the density of an object as variations in brightness.
2. Phase-microscopy is useful in clarifying details of structure and demonstrating dynamic processes in live cells.

The Differential Interference Contrast Microscope

1. A differential interference contrast (DIC) microscope makes use of a polarizing filter and a prism analyzer to accentuate phase contrast differences.
2. A DIC microscope has a greater resolution than the phase-contrast microscope, but a more shallow depth of focus at a set point.

3. The advantages of differential inter-ference contrast microscopy include production of a three-dimensional image and accentuation of phase contrast differences in unstained cells.

The Fluorescence Microscope

1. A fluorescence microscope contains special filters that emit wavelengths of ultraviolet light suitable to stimulate fluorescence in the stained specimen.

2. Special fluorescing dyes are used. If the dyes attach to the specimen, visible color is emitted and visualized.

3. Fluorescence microscopy can be used to detect the presence of infectious agents in a clinical specimen, and to observe antigen-antibody complexes.

The Transmission Electron Microscope

1. A transmission electron microscope (TEM) uses electrons and electromagnets to project images.

2. The magnification of a TEM is 100 times greater than that of a bright-field micro-scope. The resolving power is 600 times greater.

3. Specimens are dried and prepared in a special material that is sliced thinly, 1-2 Angstroms thick, for observation of cell structures.

4. The freeze-etching technique eliminates many changes in the appearance of an object, which are produced by chemical fixation, and images have a dimensional appearance.

The Scanning Electron Microscope

1. A scanning electron microscope (SEM) provides three-dimensional images of specimens that are whole.

2. An SEM has a resolving power of .010 to 0.20 μm, and a magnification of up to 100,000X.

Preparation of Materials for Bright-Field Microscopic Examination

1. Both living or dried microorganisms can be examined with a bright-field micro-scope in a stained or unstained preparation.

2. Only dried specimens can be examined with an electron microscope.

Wet and Hanging-Drop Wet Mounts

1. A simple wet mount can reveal gross morphology of larger microorganisms.

2. A hanging-drop wet mount or a culture technique is used to study motility.

3. True motility is the cellular movement from one place to another by means of flagella, cilia, or pseudopodia.

4. Brownian movement is the random jiggling motion in which the cells and particles do not travel, but instead move in response to bombardment by molecules from outside and inside the cell.

Fixed Stained Smears

1. Fixed stained smears are most useful for studying gross morphology of microorganisms.

2. Bacteria stain well with basic aniline dyes.

3. Acidic dyes have a negative charge that is repelled by the negative charges on a bacterial cell. These dyes are useful in negative stain procedures.

Simple Stains

1. Simple basic stains are often applied to heat-fixed smears to detect shape, size, and groupings of bacteria.

2. Endospores do not take up dyes readily, and stain only if special procedures are used.

Differential Stains

1. Two or more dyes are used in differential staining techniques.

2. Differences in cell wall composition or other differences are revealed by differential staining techniques.

Gram Stain

1. Gram-positive cells retain the purple primary stain, but gram-negative cells take on the red color of the counterstain.

2. Gram reactivity depends on thickness of the cell wall, pore size, and pre-sence or absence of an outer membrane.

3. Gram stains performed on young cultures are the most reliable.

Acid-Fast Stain

1. The acid-fast stain is used to diagnose the presence of the bacteria that cause tuberculosis, and developmental stages (oocysts) of fungi that cause crypto-sporidiosis in clinical specimens.

2. Acid-fast organisms and oocysts remain red even after treatment with an acid alcohol decolorizer and methylene blue counterstain.

3. In the Ziehl-Neelsen procedure, heat is required for basic carbolfuchsin to permeate walls of acid-fast organisms.

Other Differential Stains

1. The trichrome staining procedure involves a mixture of dyes for revealing protozoan structures from the background.
2. Wright's or Giemsa's stains are used for staining blood smears, and to detect spirochete bacteria, intracellular bacteria, and protozoa such as *Plasmodium* species, which cause malaria.

Special Stains

1. Bacterial flagella must be coated with chemicals and dye to increase their thickness so they can be seen with light microscopes.

2. Capsules appear as blue halos surrounding cells when a 20 percent aqueous solution of copper sulfate is applied to cells stained with crystal violet.
3. Endospores are stained with 5 percent aqueous malachite green and gentle steaming for 5 to 10 minutes.
4. A silver nitrate stain is preferred for demonstrating fungi in tissue.

Negative Stains

1. India ink or nigrosin may be used to obtain a negative stain.
2. Unstained bacteria and capsules are colorless against a dark background.
3. The advantages of negative staining are that little distortion occurs and only a bright-field microscope is required.

Study Questions for Chapter Objectives

Match an answer from column B to the item in column A. A letter may be used more than once, and some questions may be answered with two or more choices.

Column A

____ 1. Living unstained cell is white against a black background.
____ 2. Object may be a live cell in a wet mount or a dead cell in a fixed stained smear.
____ 3. Specimen is stained with fluorescent dyes.
____ 4. Specimen may be frozen, chipped off into thin sections, and coated with carbon particles.
____ 5. Specimen has a three-dimensional appearance, usually whole cells or whole objects, magnified 10,000X.
____ 6. Uses an electron beam to reveal the details of the specimen.
____ 7. Uses ultraviolet radiation to illuminate the specimen.
____ 8. Uses visible light to view the specimen.
____ 9. Living spirochete bacteria are best seen with this microscope.
____10. The highest magnification is usually 1,000X.
____11. Magnification is about 500,000X to 1,000,000X.
____12. Magnification approaches 100,000X.
____13. Resolving power is 0.01 to 0.02 μm.
____14. Resolving power is 0.002 μm.
____15. Resolving power with the 100X objective lens is 0.2 μm.
____16. Fine details of nuclear membranes, cell walls, ribosomes, and other cellular structures are seen.
____17. Bacteria are readily visible in stained or unstained preparations.
____18. A fluorescent dye attached to protein molecules is the labeled stain solution.
____19. Barrier filters protect the eyes of the observer from ultraviolet radiation.
____20. The primary microscope for observing virus structure.

Column B

a. Bright-field microscope
b. Dark-field microscope
c. Phase-contrast microscope
d. Differential interference contrast microscope
e. Fluorescence microscope
f. Transmission electron microscope
g. Scanning electron microscope

_____21. What is the correct way to represent the magnification power of a low-power objective lens?
    a. 10
    b. 10X
    c. 10 Times
    d. 40.0
    e. 40X

_____22. What is the correct way to calculate the total magnification of an object?
    a. Add the individual magnification powers of objective and ocular lenses.
    b. Multiply the magnification power of the ocular lens by 10.
    c. Multiply the magnification power of the objective lens by 10.
    d. Multiply the individual magnification powers of ocular and objective lenses.
    e. Use the magnification power of the objective lens only.

_____23. What quality of the microscope does the resolving power measure?
    a. The maximum magnification power of the microscope
    b. The minimum magnification power of the microscope
    c. The distance between the objective lens and the ocular lens
    d. The distance between the objective lens and the slide for sharp focus
    e. The minimum distance that is visible between two close objects

Match an answer from column B to the item in column A.

Column A	Column B
_____24. Name for microscope lens you look through	a. Substage lamp
_____25. Lens placed over the object	b. Objective lens
_____26. Regulates the light intensity	c. Pinion knob
_____27. Provides illumination	d. Ocular lens
_____28. Raises and lowers condenser lens	e. Iris diaphragm

Write in the answers in the table below:

	Color of Positive Result	Color of Negative Result
Gram stain	29._____	30._____
Acid-fast stain	31._____	32._____

Write the name and the time or method of application of each solution used in the Gram stain procedure in the correct order in which the solutions are used.

33. _____Application time _____

34. _____Application time _____

35. _____Application method _____

    _____

36. _____Application time _____

Write the name and the time or method of application of each solution used in the Ziehl-Neelsen acid-fast stain procedure in the correct order in which the solutions are used.

37. _____Application time _____

38. _____Application method _____

    _____

39. _____Application time _____

40. Define simple stain procedure.

_____

_____

_____

41. Define differential stain procedure.

_____

_____

_____

Write the letter *A* next to the acidic dyes and the letter *B* next to the basic dyes in the following list. Then write "cell" next to the dye that stains the cell, and "background" next to the dye that does not stain the cell.

42. Eosin _____

43. Crystal violet _____

44. Nigrosin _____

45. Acidic fuchsin _____

46. Safranin _____

47. Methylene blue _____

48. Basic carbolfuchsin _____

49. In a brief essay, explain why acidic dyes stain the background, and basic dyes stain the cell.

_____

_____

_____

_____

Write the type of microscope that is used to observe each of the following:

50. Causative agent of syphilis live and unstained: _____

51. Cytoplasmic streaming: _____

52. Surface 3-D view of a bacterium: _____

53. An antigen-antibody combination: _____

54. Dynamic state of organelles: _____

55. Phagocytosis: _____

56. Structure of viruses: _____

57. Budding of yeast cells: _____

58. Ameba in three dimensions: _____

59. Wright-stained human blood: _____

60. Fluorescent-stained rabies virus: _____

61. The Gram stain detects two main kinds of bacteria, based on differences in the characteristics of the cell wall. Explain these differences.

_____

_____

_____

_____

_____

_____

62. Define the word mordant. Identify the mordant in the Gram stain.

_____

_____

_____

_____

63. Identify the decolorizer in the Gram stain. _____

64. Identify the decolorizer in the Ziehl-Neelsen acid-fast stain.

_____

65. Define the word counterstain.

_____

_____

66. Identify the counterstain in the Gram stain. _____

67. Identify the counterstain in the Ziehl-Neelsen acid-fast stain. _____

____68. Staining procedures in which the cells are colorless against a colored background
are called:
a. Negative stain
b. Positive stain
c. Basic dye
d. Differential stain
e. Simple stain

69. Why is proper illumination so important in making accurate microscopic observations?
How can the light intensity be regulated?

_____

_____

_____

_____

70. What is the most critical step in the Gram stain? Why?

_____

_____

_____

71. What is the primary stain in the Gram stain? _____

In the Ziehl-Neelsen acid-fast stain? _____

72. Name two advantages associated with the use of negative stains.

_____

_____

_____

73. Describe briefly how you could demonstrate Brownian movement or cytoplasmic streaming in the laboratory.

_____

_____

_____

_____

74. If one student obtained gram-negative bacilli, and another obtained gram-positive bacilli from the same culture, how could you explain the results?

_____

_____

_____

_____

75. Explain the need for the variety of stains described in this chapter.

_____

_____

_____

_____

CHAPTER 4

Structure of Microbial Cells

Learning Objectives

1. Describe the major differences between procaryotes and eucaryotes.
2. Differentiate between the cell walls of gram-positive and gram-negative bacteria.
3. Describe the significance of the outer membrane of gram-negative bacteria.
4. Explain passive and active transport of molecules across plasma membranes.
5. Explain the significance of bacterial endospores.
6. List the membranous organelles of eucaryotes.

Study Outline

Procaryotes

1. Procaryotes lack membrane-bound organelles.
2. All the bacteria are procaryotes.

Shapes, Sizes, and Arrangements of Procaryotic Cells

1. Most bacterial cells are either rod-shaped (bacilli), spherical (cocci), or spiral-shaped (spirilla).
2. Bacteria are usually 0.2 to 1.5 μm in diameter and 1.0 to 6.0 μm long.
3. Cellular arrangements can be in pairs (diplo-), chains (strepto-), palisades, packets, or clusters (staphylo-).

Cell Surface Structures

1. All bacteria, except mycoplasmas, have cell walls.
2. Cell walls provide support and protection.

Glycocalyx

1. The glycocalyx is a capsule of polysaccharides, or a slime layer of glycoproteins outside the cell wall.

2. Encapsulated strains of *Streptococcus pneumoniae, Haemophilus influenzae,* and *Neisseria meningitis* cause serious diseases.

Cell Wall

1. Cell walls maintain the rigid shapes of bacteria.
2. Bacterial cell walls contain a unique chemical known as peptidoglycan.
3. Peptidoglycan contains two derivatives of glucose (N-acetylglucosamine, or NAG, and N-acetylmuramic acid, or NAM) and amino acids.

The Cell Wall of Gram-Positive Bacteria

1. Peptidoglycan makes up 90 percent of the cell walls in gram-positive bacteria.
2. Teichoic acids contribute to the stability of the cell walls.
3. Mycolic acids in cell walls of *Mycobacterium tuberculosis* make that organism difficult to stain.

The Cell Wall of Gram-Negative Bacteria

1. Peptidoglycan makes up 5 to 10 percent of the cell walls in gram-negative bacteria.
2. All gram-negative bacteria have outer membranes of proteins, phospholipids, and lipopolysaccharides.
3. The lipopolysaccharide layer of the outer membrane acts as an endotoxin when released at cell death.

The Cell Wall in Cell Division

1. The cell wall participates in cell growth and division.
2. An infolding of the cell wall allows newly- synthesized cell wall material to be deposited midway in a cell.

Surface Appendages

1. Appendages of procaryotes allow them to move and to adhere to solid surfaces.
2. Special staining techniques are required to view appendages.

Flagella

1. Some bacteria have long, filamentous appendages, known as flagella, for locomotion.
2. Flagella are made of proteins known as flagellin and are attached by flexible hooks and basal bodies to the cell.

Axial Filaments

1. Spirochetes have axial filaments that wind around the organisms between an outer sheath and the outer cytoplasm.
2. *Treponema pallidum* is an organism that moves by means of axial filaments.

Pili (Fimbriae)

1. Pili are short, fine appendages that surround some bacteria and allow them to adhere to epithelial surfaces.
2. Sex pili have a role in the transfer of DNA from one bacterium to another during conjugation.

Plasma (Cytoplasmic) Membrane

1. The plasma membrane is composed of proteins embedded in two layers of phospholipids.
2. Portions of the lipid molecules alternate between a rigid and a fluid state.

The Plasma Membrane as a Barrier

1. The plasma membrane regulates movement of molecules entering or leaving cells.
2. Transfer of molecules across membranes is limited by size and solubility of molecules, availability of carrier molecules, and sufficient quantities of energy.
3. Molecules move across membranes by passive transport in diffusion, facilitated diffusion, and osmosis.
4. Active transport of molecules across membranes requires ATP or other available phosphate.

The Membrane and Chemical Activity

1. The plasma membrane is the site of ATP-generating reactions.
2. Structural components of cells are also synthesized by the plasma membrane.
3. Photosynthetic pigments are found on plasma membranes.

The Plasma Membrane in Secretion

1. Hydrolytic enzymes, toxins, and products that interfere with antibody activity are secreted through plasma membranes.
2. These products are necessary for survival of the cell.

Cytoplasm

1. Cytoplasm of procaryotes contains water, carbohydrates, proteins, lipids, and inorganic salts.
2. Internal membranes of procaryotes have the same chemical composition as the plasma membrane.

Granules

1. Poly-β-hydroxybutyric acid (PHB) is stored in granules of many procaryotes.
2. Other materials stored in granules are glycogen, sulfur, and inorganic phosphates.

Ribosomes

1. Ribosomes are composed of RNA and protein; they are the location for protein synthesis.
2. The procaryotic ribosome is 70S with two subunits: one of 30S and one of 50S.

Nucleoid

1. The nucleoid is the region where DNA, the hereditary molecule, is found.
2. The nucleoid is not surrounded by a membrane.

Plasmids

1. Some bacteria have small circular molecules of DNA that are independent of the nucleoid known as plasmids.

2. Plasmids replicate independently and are transferable under special circumstances.

Endospores

1. An endospore is the multilayered dormant stage in the life cycle of species of *Bacillus* and *Clostridium*.

2. Spores are resistant to heat, cold, radiation, and disinfectants.

3. Heat and an environment that supports growth activates spores to germinate, producing one cell.

Eucaryotes

1. Eucaryotic cells are larger and more complex structurally than procaryotic cells.

2. Algae, protozoa, and fungi make up the microbial eucaryotes.

Shapes, Sizes, and Arrangements of Eucaryotic Cells

1. Algae vary in size from microscopic forms to seaweeds that reach 100 m in length.

2. Protozoa are unicellular organisms that vary in size from 1.0 µm to more than 250 µm.

3. Motile, feeding stages of protozoa are called trophozoites.

4. Nonmotile, feeding stages of protozoa are known as cysts.

5. Fungi include unicellular yeasts and multicellular molds.

Cell-Surface Structures

1. Algae and fungi have cell walls that surround a plasma membrane, and protozoa have a plasma membrane, or pellicle, as their outer boundary.

2. The cell walls are largely protective, but also function in maintaining rigid shapes.

Cell Wall

1. Cell walls of fungi contain cellulose, or chitin.

2. Silica, cellulose, polysaccharides, and proteins are constituents of algal cell walls.

3. Cell walls of eucaryotes contain no peptidoglycan.

Surface Appendages

1. Most protozoa and some algae are motile during at least one stage of their development.

2. Some protozoa have temporary extensions of cytoplasm, called pseudopodia, that transport the cell.

3. Other protozoa have appendages such as flagella or cilia for motility.

Flagella

1. Some protozoa and algae move by means of flagella.

2. Each flagellum has a peripheral ring of nine double microtubules and two central microtubules, a "9 + 2" pattern.

Cilia

1. One group of protozoa move by means of cilia.

2. Cilia have the same "9 + 2" pattern of microtubules as flagella.

Plasma (Cytoplasmic) Membrane

1. The plasma membrane of eucaryotes is similar to that of procaryotes, except that it contains sterols.

2. Molecules move across plasma membranes by passive and active transport mechanisms.

3. Two processes of active transport found in eucaryotes, but not in procaryotes, are endocytosis and exocytosis.

Cytoplasm

1. The cytoplasm of eucaryotic cells is a mixture of organic and inorganic materials.

2. The flowing movement of eucaryotic cytoplasm is known as cytoplasmic streaming.

Internal Membranes

1. Endoplasmic reticulum (er) is a network of internal membranes in eucaryote cells.

2. The passageways of the endoplasmic reticulum provide a type of chemical transport system within a cell. Phospholipids are synthesized on these membranes.

3. Ribosomes are attached to portions of the endoplasmic reticulum, making it appear "rough" or bumpy on electron micro-graphs. This appearance is known as rough er.

Granules

1. Granules of eucaryotic cells contain polysaccharides and lipids.

2. The solidifying agent, agar, is a polysaccharide derived from a red marine alga.

Vacuoles

1. Vacuoles contain fluids, soluble materials, and particulate material.
2. Protozoan vacuoles aid in excreting excess water and in food gathering.

Vesicles

1. Infoldings of the plasma membrane are called vesicles. The infolding occurs in the process of endocytosis or exocytosis.
2. Vesicles are temporary structures that form on the surface of phagocytic cells.

Ribosomes

1. Eucaryotic ribosomes have an 80S value with two subunits: one of 60S and one of 40S.
2. Smaller ribosomes are found in mitochondria and chloroplasts.
3. Ribosomes are the sites of protein synthesis.

Mitochondria

1. Mitochondria are submicroscopic structures enclosed by two layers of membrane. Infoldings of the inner membranes are called cristae.
2. Mitochondria are sites of respiration and fatty-acid synthesis.
3. Energy released during respiration reactions is conserved in energy-rich bonds, resulting in the nickname "power house."
4. The protein-synthesizing systems of mitochondria are unlike those found in procaryotes or eucaryotes.
5. The membranes and ribosomes resemble those of procaryotic cells.
6. A mitochondrion has a unique DNA molecule that replicates independently of the nuclear DNA. The mitochondrion replicates itself independently of the replication of nuclear DNA.

Chloroplasts

1. Chloroplasts are usually green-colored structures with a two-layered outer membrane; inner membranes are called thylakoids.
2. Chemical reactions of photosynthesis occur in the chloroplasts of algae.
3. Thylakoids possess chlorophyll pigments and enzymes required for photosynthesis.
4. Chloroplasts contain DNA and ribosomes.

5. Ribosomes of chloroplasts and bacteria are almost identical.

The Golgi Complex

1. The Golgi complex consists of narrowly stacked membranes, the cisternae, which are surrounded by vesicles.
2. The Golgi complex modifies and packages complex structural molecules, which contain lipids, proteins, and carbohydrates, and transports them to other parts of the cell.

Lysosomes

1. Lysosomes are membranous sacs that contain digestive enzymes.
2. Lysosomes fuse with vacuoles, or vesicles formed by endocytosis, and lysosomal enzymes digest the engulfed particles and cells.

Cytoskeleton

1. The cytoskeleton participates in cell movement and in cell division.
2. The cytoskeleton of eucaryotic cells is made up of microtubules of a protein called tubulin, and microfilaments of actin protein.
3. Tubulin alternates between an assembled and a disassembled state in different stages of the cell cycle. Actin is a contractile protein that provides flexibility in intracellular movements.

Nucleus

1. Chromosomes contain DNA and histone proteins; they are found in a membrane-bound organelle known as the nucleus.
2. Small dark-staining bodies known as nucleoli contain RNA. These bodies are observed in some nuclei.
3. Some DNA is complexed with histones to form nucleosomes.
4. Strands of complexed and naked DNA are called chromatin.

Plasmids

1. Some yeast cells contain plasmids.
2. The DNA of plasmids may or may not be subject to chromosomal regulation.

Cysts

1. Some protozoa form dormant stages called cysts when environmental conditions are unfavorable.
2. Cysts are susceptible to heat and drying, but are resistant to cold.
3. A trophozite is the actively motile feeding cell that emerges from a cyst under favorable conditions.

Study Questions for Chapter Objectives

Identify the following structures as parts of eucaryotic cells, by writing E next to the structure, or as parts of procaryotic cells, by writing P next to the structure. If the structure is found in both cell types, write both P and E.

____ 1. Nucleus

____ 2. Ribosome

____ 3. Mitochondrion

____ 4. Chloroplast

____ 5. Endospore

____ 6. Glycocalyx

____ 7. Cilia

____ 8. Cristae

____ 9. Thylakoid

____10. Periplasm

____11. Cyst

____12. Endoplasmic reticulum

____13. Golgi complex

____14. Lysosome

____15. Nucleolus

____16. Microtubule

____17. Nucleoid

____18. Pili

____19. Flagella

____20. Vesicle

____21. Cytoskeleton

____22. Contractile vacuole

____23. Chromosome

____24. Plasma membrane

Write the name of the structures numbered 25 to 32 in this cross-sectional diagram of a procaryotic cell.

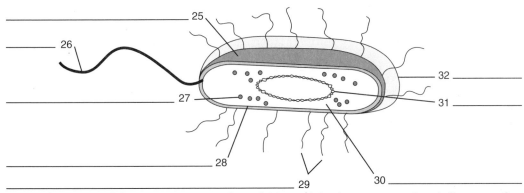

Write the name of the structures numbered 33 to 49 in the cross-sectional diagram of a eucaryotic cell.

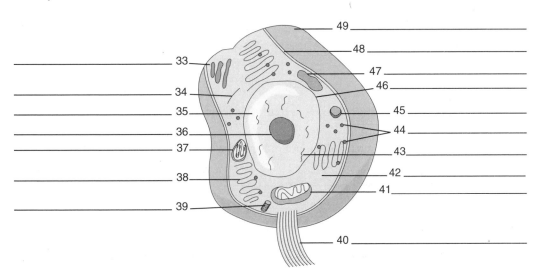

Refer to the diagram for questions 25 to 32, which illustrates the structures of a procaryotic cell. Write in a function for each structure below.

50. Function of 25: _____

51. Function of 26: _____

52. Function of 27: _____

53. Function of 28: _____

54. Function of 29: _____

55. Function of 30: _____

56. Function of 31: _____

57. Function of 32: _____

Match the chemical nature in column B to the structures of a procaryotic cell in column A.

Column A	Column B
___58. Nucleoid	a. Polysaccharides
___59. Capsule	b. Protein, water, carbohydrates, lipids, inorganic salts
___60. Flagellum	c. Protein
___61. Cell wall	d. Phospholipids, proteins
___62. Plasma membrane	e. Peptidoglycan, teichoic acid
___63. Ribosome	f. Proteins, RNA
___64. Cytoplasm	g. DNA

Write in the name of the membranous organelle of eucaryotic cells with the function given below:

65. Contains chromosomes: _____

66. Packages proteins, lipids, and carbohydrates: _____

67. Contains digestive enzymes: _____

68. Carries out fatty-acid synthesis and respiration reactions that form energy-rich

    molecules: _____

69. Forms temporarily to take in or discharge materials from the cell: _____

70. Contains fluids and soluble and particulate material, which is brought into the cell

    by endocytosis: _____

71. Contains photosynthetic pigments: _____

    _____

72. Explain how the cell walls of gram-negative bacteria differ from the cell walls of gram-positive bacteria.

_____

_____

_____

_____

_____

_____

_____

73. Explain passive and active transport of molecules across the plasma membrane.

_____

_____

_____

_____

_____

74. What is the significance of the outer membrane of gram-negative bacteria?

_____

_____

75. What word describes bacterial endospores relative to heating, drying, radiation, dyes, and disinfectants? _____

76. How might this property (see question 75) of bacterial endospores influence the commercial canning of vegetables, such as green beans and peas, which may contain bacterial spores from the soil?

_____

_____

Quantitative Relationships

Write *a* if choice *a* is larger or of greater magnitude than *b*.

Write *b* if choice *b* is larger or of greater magnitude than *a*.

Write *c* if both *a* and *b* are about the same, or if neither applies.

_____77. The length and width of the flagella:
   a. Procaryote
   b. Eucaryote

_____78. Mass of the ribosome:
   a. Procaryote
   b. Eucaryote

_____79. Cell membrane has both phospholipids and proteins:
   a. Procaryote
   b. Eucaryote

_____80. Peptidoglycan layer:
   a. Gram-positive cell
   b. Gram-negative cell

GROWTH, METABOLISM, AND VARIATION

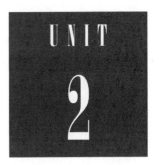

UNIT

2

CHAPTER

5

Microbial Growth

Learning Objectives

1. Define "generation time."
2. Identify the phases of growth on a population-growth curve.
3. Explain why logarithmic growth is rarely encountered in nature.
4. Classify microorganisms according to energy and carbon sources.
5. Describe conditions that must be met in the laboratory in order to culture microorganisms.
6. Describe three methods for obtaining isolated colonies of bacteria.
7. Contrast the advantages and disadvantages of direct and indirect estimations of bacterial numbers.

Study Outline

Introduction

1. The time required for microbial growth and reproduction is known as the "generation time."
2. The generation time of procaryotes is usually shorter than that of eucaryotes.

The Population-Growth Curve

1. The term "growth" in microbiology is usually applied to populations.
2. Four phases of a population-growth curve can be demonstrated in the laboratory.

The Lag Phase

1. A lag phase occurs when microorganisms are transferred to a fresh culture medium.

2. The number of organisms does not increase noticeably during the lag phase but the cells are metabolically active.

The Logarithmic or Exponential Phase

1. During the logarithmic or exponential phase, the rate of population growth is constant with time.

2. Logarithmic growth rarely occurs in nature because microorganisms do not occur in pure culture and optimal growth conditions cannot be sustained for long periods.

The Stationary Phase

1. During the stationary phase, which may last for a few hours to several days, the total number of viable cells remains constant.

2. Growth is inhibited when an essential nutrient is limited, or when products of metabolism accumulate.

The Death Phase

1. In the death phase, the number of viable cells decreases exponentially with time.

2. The death phase continues until most, if not all, microorganisms are dead.

Significance of a Population-Growth Curve

1. Microorganisms are most active metabolically during the logarithmic phase.

2. An understanding of growth kinetics is important in industrial fermentations.

Factors Influencing Microbial Growth

1. Some microorganisms can tolerate extreme environmental conditions, while others exhibit limitations.

2. The expansion of microbial populations is controlled by changing environmental conditions and competition for nutrients.

Temperature

1. Microorganisms are classified as thermophiles, mesophiles, or psychrophiles according to temperature requirements.

2. A majority of human pathogens grow best at body temperature.

Water

1. Some microorganisms die quickly in the absence of water.

2. Transport media prevent the drying of clinical specimens on swabs.

Osmotic Pressure

1. Optimal growth of microorganisms is obtained when solute concentrations in the cell and environment are isotonic.

2. Microorganisms that can grow in the presence of excess solutes are called osmotolerant.

Salinity

1. Obligate halophiles (salt-loving microorganisms) are found in saline lakes and basins, and in oceans.

2. Facultative halophiles can tolerate concentrations of NaCl up to 10 percent.

Hydrostatic Pressure

1. Most microorganisms are inhibited by hydrostatic pressure of 200 to 600 atmospheres. Organisms found in the deepest oceans are barophiles.

2. Microorganisms that survive under conditions of increased hydrostatic pressure are called barotolerant.

Atmospheric Conditions

1. Obligate aerobes require oxygen gas for growth.

2. Obligate anaerobes grow only in the absence of oxygen.

3. Facultative anaerobes grow with or without oxygen.

4. Microaerophilic organisms require less oxygen than that found in the atmosphere.

5. Capneic bacteria need carbon dioxide in concentrations greater than that found in the atmosphere.

pH

1. Almost all microorganisms grow best at a pH that approximates neutrality; some grow very well in highly acidic environments.

2. The pH of culture media is controlled by adding buffers.

Light Intensity

1. High intensities of ultraviolet (UV) and visible light may be detrimental to cells.

2. Damaging free radicals are formed when cytochromes and flavins absorb visible light in large quantities.

Nutritional Requirements

1. Microorganisms get energy from the sun or from chemical compounds.

2. Phototrophs derive energy from the sun, and chemotrophs derive energy from chemical sources.

Carbon

1. Autotrophic bacteria obtain carbon from carbon dioxide.
2. Heterotrophic organisms depend on organic carbon compounds and CO_2.

Nitrogen

1. All life forms require nitrogen to build amino acids, proteins, and other molecules.
2. Some microorganisms obtain nitrogen from proteins and polypeptides, while others use nitrogen from inorganic sources or from atmospheric nitrogen gas.

Sulfur and Phosphorus

1. Inorganic salts of sulfates, sulfides, and thiosulfates, and some amino acids, are common sources of sulfur for microorganisms.
2. The requirement for phosphorus can be met by phosphorus-containing inorganic or organic compounds.

Other Minerals

1. Microorganisms require certain minerals in trace amounts.
2. Minerals such as magnesium (Mg), molybdenum (Mo), manganese (Mn), iron (Fe), and zinc (Zn) activate many enzyme reactions.

Growth Factors

1. Vitamins, amino acids, pyrimidines, purines, porphyrins, and other growth factors must be supplied if an organism does not synthesize them in sufficient amounts.
2. The need for specific growth factors is the basis of many microbiological assays.

Cultivation of Microorganisms in the Laboratory

1. Substances that support the growth of microorganisms are called media.
2. Microorganisms may be grown in the laboratory on synthetic defined media in which all components and their quantities are known.
3. Microorganisms may be grown in the laboratory on complex media that have components of unknown and inexact composition, such as yeast extract.

Liquid, Semisolid, and Solid Media

1. Culture media may be liquid, semisolid, or solid and may be dispensed in tubes, bottles, or Petri plates.
2. Semisolid and solid media contain agar or gelatin as solidifying agents.

Selective and Differential Media

1. Dyes, salts, or antimicrobial agents can be added to media to make them selective for a particular group of microorganisms.
2. A specific substrate, a pH indicator, dyes, or salts in media differentiate colonies by their metabolic types.

Pure Culture Techniques

1. Pure colonies can be obtained by preparing streak, pour, or spread plates.
2. Pure cultures are useful to identify microorganisms.

Special Culture Techniques

1. Special culture techniques are used to grow viruses, rickettsias, protozoa, and helminths.
2. Viruses produce specific cytopathic effects (CPE) in host cells.

Animal Inoculation

1. Guinea pigs and mice are used to confirm the pathogenicity of some bacteria, viruses, and fungi.
2. Some pathogens, such as those causing leprosy and syphilis, have not been grown successfully outside the animal body.

Continuous and Synchronized Cultures

1. Continuous culture techniques may be employed to produce large numbers of microorganisms or to recover specific metabolites.
2. Synchronized cultures permit the study of details of cell cycles.

Continuous Culture

1. A growth chamber called the chemostat allows regular additions of fresh nutrients and removal of spent media, in a continuous open culture system.
2. Cells remain in one phase, such as the logarithmic phase.

Synchronized Culture

1. Growth of a microbial population can be inhibited by a reduction in temperature or the deprivation of an essential nutrient; when growth requirements are restored, cell division is synchronized.
2. Cells may divide synchronously if all cells are in the same stage of a cell cycle; this is accomplished by filtering a culture to collect cells of a single size.

Methods of Measuring Growth

1. Milk, food, and drinking water must meet quantitative and qualitative standards for microorganisms.
2. Measurements of cell mass or cell numbers provide quantitative information.

Measurements of Cell Mass

1. Measurements of cell mass may be obtained by weighing, turbidimetric, or chemical methods.
2. These methods do not distinguish between live and dead cells.

Measurement of Cell Weight

1. Dry weight measurements are more accurate than wet weight measurements.
2. Measurements of dry weight are time-consuming and only suitable for massive populations of cells.

Turbidimetric Measurement

1. Visible turbidity in a liquid medium can be measured in a spectrophotometer in optical density (O.D.) or percent transmittance (%T) units.
2. The O.D. is proportional to cell mass between 0.01 mg and 0.5 mg dry weight.

Chemical Analysis

1. Amounts of particular components in a microbial population are proportional to cell mass.

2. The nitrogen content is often measured to assess biomass.

Measurement of Cell Number

1. Microscopy and electronic devices provide direct estimations of total number of cells.
2. Viable numbers of cells can be determined by a culture technique.

Direct Cell Counts

1. The number of cells in a suspension can be counted microscopically in special counting chambers, or by electronic counting devices.
2. Direct microscopic and electronic counts do not differentiate between live and dead cells.

Viable Cell Counts

1. Numbers of viable bacteria can be determined by using serial dilutions of samples of water, milk, food, or soil.
2. The agar plate that contains between 30 to 300 colonies is counted; the colony count is multiplied by the dilution factor to obtain the number of colony-forming units (CFU) per ml.

Indirect Measurements

1. Reduction of methylene blue is the basis for determining relative numbers of bacteria for grading milk.
2. Quantitative determinations of chemical products are proportional to the density of a bacterial population under carefully controlled conditions.

 Study Questions for Chapter Objectives

Match the statements in column A with a letter in column B:

Column A

_____1. Carbon dioxide and light energy are required.
_____2. Organic carbon molecules and light energy are required.
_____3. Carbon dioxide and inorganic chemicals are required. Light is not required.
_____4. Organic carbon molecules and other chemicals are required. Light is not required.
_____5. An organism grows if CO_2, minerals, water, and light are provided.
_____6. An organism grows if a variety of organic compounds, minerals, vitamins, and water are provided.
_____7. An organism will grow if light and organic compounds are provided.
_____8. An organism grows if CO_2, minerals, and water are provided.

Column B

a. Chemoheterotroph
b. Photoheterotroph
c. Chemoautotroph
d. Photoautotroph

POPULATION–GROWTH CURVE EXERCISE:

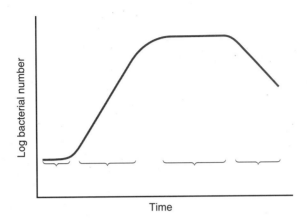

9. Color the lag phase with a blue pencil, and write "lag phase" on the correct portion of the graph.
10. Color the logarithmic phase with a green pencil, and write "log phase" on the correct portion of the graph.
11. Color the stationary phase yellow, and write "stationary phase" on the correct portion of the graph.
12. Color the death phase red, and write "death phase" on the correct portion of the graph.

Use the population-growth curve above to match a letter in column B to a statement in column A:

Column A	Column B
___13. Total number of viable cells remains constant.	a. Lag
___14. Number of dead cells outnumbers viable cells.	b. Logarithmic
___15. Bacteria adjust to new medium.	c. Stationary
___16. Rate of cells dying equals rate of cells dividing.	d. Death
___17. Cells are not dividing, and nutrients are plentiful.	
___18. Medium is depleted of nutrients; live population decreases rapidly.	
___19. Medium is depleted of nutrients, and live population stays constant.	
___20. Acids and other wasteproducts accumulate, cells divide slowly, stable live population count.	
___21. Low population count, little or no waste products.	
___22. Low population count increases rapidly to a high count.	
___23. Depletion of nutrients causes cells to be small; population is constant.	
___24. Binary fission occurs at the fastest rate.	

25. Define "generation time."

_____

_____

26. Generation time is calculated for the actively-dividing cells found in which phase of growth? _____

Briefly describe three methods for the isolation of colonies on a nutrient agar medium.

27. _____

_____

_____

28. _____

_____

_____

29. _____

_____

_____

Identify two points in order to explain why logarithmic growth of bacterial cells is rarely encountered in nature.

30. _____

_____

31. _____

_____

List nine environmental factors to be considered for the successful cultivation of a micro-organism in the laboratory.

32. _____ 37. _____

33. _____ 38. _____

34. _____ 39. _____

35. _____ 40. _____

36. _____

41. Describe briefly the environmental factors and nutrients that would be necessary for the laboratory cultivation of a chemoheterotrophic thermophilic anaerobic bacteria obtained from a soil compost pile.

_____

_____

_____

_____

42. Name three methods used to determine cell mass. List an advantage and a disadvantage of these methods.

_____

_____

_____

_____

_____

_____

43. Name four methods used to determine cell number. List an advantage and a disadvantage of these methods.

_____

_____

_____

_____

_____

_____

_____

_____

6 Microbial Metabolism and Regulation

Learning Objectives

1. Differentiate between catabolic and anabolic reactions.
2. Recognize the six types of enzyme-catalyzed reactions.
3. Identify the three major pathways in aerobic respiration and their roles in generating ATP.
4. Contrast the efficiency of aerobic respiration, fermentation, and anaerobic respiration in metabolism.
5. List the final electron acceptors of aerobes and anaerobes.
6. Identify one or more roles of ATP in metabolism.
7. Describe four mechanisms that control microbial metabolism.

Study Outline

Energy Resources

1. The energy required to generate ATP is derived from chemical compounds in chemotrophs and from the sun in phototrophs.
2. Energy is released as bonds of chemical compounds are broken.

Role of Enzymes

1. Enzymes catalyze metabolic reactions upon specific molecules called substrates.
2. The product of a reaction may be the substrate for another enzyme.

Classification of Enzymes

1. Enzymes are categorized into six classes, according to the type of reaction catalyzed.
2. Oxidoreductases catalyze transfer of electrons of hydrogen (H).
   $$AH_2 + B \rightleftharpoons A + BH_2$$
3. Transferases catalyze transfer of functional groups (R).
   $$AR + B \rightleftharpoons BR + A$$

4. Hydrolases catalyze the breaking of chemical bonds in the presence of water
   $$AB + H_2O \rightleftharpoons AOH + BH$$
5. Lyases catalyze removal or addition of functional groups.
   $$AR \rightleftharpoons A + R$$
6. Isomerases catalyze rearrangement of atoms within a molecule.
   $$AB \rightleftharpoons BA$$
7. Ligases catalyze the formation of bonds of polymers, with energy derived from ATP.
   $$A + B + ATP \rightleftharpoons AB + ADP + Pi$$
8. Exoenzymes act on substrates outside the cell, and endoenzymes act on substrates within the cell.

Naming of Enzymes

1. Enzymes are named according to the type of reaction that is catalyzed and the name of the substrate acted upon.
2. The suffix *ase* is used.

Coenzymes and Essential Ions

1. Coenzymes are organic molecules that are not protein; they participate in some enzyme reactions.
2. Adenosine triphosphate (ATP), flavin adenine dinucleotide (FAD), and nicotinamide adenine dinucleotide (NAD) are examples of coenzymes.
3. Certain metal ions are required for optimal activity of some phosphatases and peptidases.

Factors Influencing the Rate of Enzyme Reactions

1. The rate at which enzyme reactions proceed is influenced by environmental factors.
2. Rates of enzyme reactions may also be determined by the presence of specific accelerating or inhibiting factors.

pH

1. The pH of the cellular environment affects affinities of enzymes for their substrates.
2. Reaction rates are most rapid at an optimal pH.

Temperature

1. The rate of chemical reactions is increased at higher temperatures, but excessive exposure to heat inactivates enzymes by denaturation.
2. Excessive exposure to cold interferes with the activity of enzymes, but not with their structural integrity.

Substrate Concentration

1. Increased concentrations of substrate increase the rate of a reaction until active sites on the enzyme are saturated.
2. The lowest concentration of substrate to yield one-half maximum velocity is the most efficient.

Enzyme Concentration

1. With a fixed amount of substrate, as the enzyme concentration is increased, the reaction rate increases.
2. The reaction rate levels off as substrate is bound to active sites of the enzyme.

Product Concentration

1. An accumulation of products causes reversal of a single-step reaction.
2. If the products of an enzyme's action become substrates in other reactions, the enzyme continues to convert substrate to product.

Inhibiting Substances

1. Inhibitors can bind to an enzyme in a reversible or irreversible manner.
2. Competitive inhibition by a structurally-similar substrate is reversible when the substrate level is increased.
3. Noncompetitive inhibition causes a conformational change in an enzyme so it cannot bind with its substrate.

Catabolism: Energy-Generating Reactions

1. Microbial cells generate ATP by respiration, fermentation, or photosynthesis.
2. All cells liberate energy from nutrients by respiration; some cells release energy by fermentation of nutrients.

Respiration

1. During respiration, electrons are transferred to a final electron acceptor that is an inorganic molecule.
2. Many microorganisms use oxygen as the final electron acceptor in aerobic respiration; other microorganisms that cannot use oxygen use other inorganic molecules as final electron acceptors in anaerobic respiration.

Aerobic Respiration

1. ATP is generated in aerobic microorganisms by three pathways: 1) glycolysis, 2) the citric acid cycle, and 3) the electron transport chain.
2. Nutrients are oxidized to CO_2, and molecular oxygen is reduced to H_2O.

Glycolysis

1. Glycolysis occurs in a series of reactions called the Embden-Meyerhof-Parnas Pathway (EMP).
2. Glucose is converted to two molecules of pyruvic acid, with a net production of two molecules of ATP by substrate phos- phorylation, and two molecules of reduced NAD.

The Metabolic Bridge

1. The major chemical pathways in cells are often connected by reactions that may be called metabolic bridges.
2. The metabolic bridge between glycolysis and the citric acid cycle is a reaction that oxidizes pyruvic acid and produces CO_2, acetyl-CoA, and NADH.

The Citric Acid Cycle

1. The citric acid cycle is a series of reactions that liberate energy from citric acid.
2. The following are produced per turn of the citric acid cycle: three molecules of CO_2, three molecules of NADH, one molecule of FADH, and one molecule of guanosine triphosphate (GTP), which is converted to ATP.

The Electron Transport Chain

1. The electron transport chain consists of carrier molecules that transport electrons to a final electron acceptor.
2. Protons are pumped across the membrane and establish a proton gradient. As protons move back into the cell, ATP is generated by oxidative phosphorylation.

Tallying the Score of Energy Yields

1. The complete oxidation of a molecule of glucose yields 38 molecules of ATP in procaryotes.
2. Aerobic respiration yields 36 molecules of ATP in eucaryotes.

Anaerobic Respiration

1. Obligated anaerobes lack the enzymes necessary to release all of the potential energy from glucose; oxygen is toxic to strict anaerobes.
2. Anaerobic microorganisms use inorganic molecules such as CO_2, NO_3^- (nitrate ion), or SO_4^{2-} (sulfate ion) as final electron acceptors.

Fermentation

1. Pyruvic acid may be converted by fermentation to a variety of products to oxidize the two molecules of reduced NAD.
2. When oxygen is unavailable, some facultatively anaerobic organisms obtain energy by this process.

Metabolism of Other Carbohydrates, Lipids, and Proteins

1. Other sugars, besides glucose, may be used as an energy source.
2. Large polymeric molecules, such as starch and proteins, are broken down to monomeric units, such as sugars and amino-acids, respectively, which enter metabolic pathways.

Photosynthesis

1. The process of photosynthesis in cyanobacteria, most algae, plants, and some bacteria converts light energy to chemical energy.
2. Plants, cyanobacteria, and algae employ H_2O as the source of hydrogens and electrons, and they release oxygen.
3. In anaerobic conditions, some phototrophic bacteria use other reduced organic or inorganic compounds as a source of electrons.
4. The overall reaction for photosynthesis can be expressed as follows:

   $$CO_2 + 2H_2X \xrightarrow{\text{light}} (CH_2O) + 2X + H_2O$$

5. Light energy is absorbed by chlorophyll or another pigment and transferred to a reaction center, releasing an electron.
6. The pattern of electron flow differs in anoxygenic and oxygenic photosynthesis.
7. Production of an ATP from ADP and inorganic phosphate with energy from light-stimulated reactions is photophosphorylation.

Anabolism: Energy-Requiring Reactions

1. Autotrophs fix CO_2 as the sole source of carbon, and heterotrophs may use CO_2 but require an organic carbon source.
2. ATP and reducing power, required in all synthetic pathways, are supplied by photosynthesis, respiration, or fermentation.

Synthesis of Carbohydrates

1. The major product of CO_2-fixation in autotrophs is glyceric acid phosphate.
2. Intermediates of the Calvin-Benson cycle either enter polysaccharide synthetic pathways or the Embden-Meyerhof pathway.
3. The synthesis of polysaccharides requires ATP and a primer that consists of a polysaccharide or a protein.

Synthesis of Proteins

1. Synthesis of proteins is dependent on the availability of amino acids.
2. Carbon skeletons of most amino acids are derived from organic acid intermediates of glycolysis or the citric acid cycle.

Synthesis of Lipids

1. Microorganisms incorporate fatty acids of the environment, or those that are synthesized from acetyl-CoA, into phospholipids of the cell membranes.

2. The major energy reserve of bacteria, poly-β-hydroxybutyric acid, is a product in fatty acid synthesis or of pyruvic acid fermentation.

Integration of Catabolism and Anabolism

1. Catabolic and anabolic pathways are usually distinct, but they are linked by key metabolites and the ATP-ADP system.

2. Biochemical pathways that participate in catabolic and anabolic reactions are called amphibolic pathways.

Control Mechanisms for Metabolism

1. At least one thousand interdependent reactions occur in the single compartment of a procaryotic cell.

2. A certain amount of regulation is obtained in eucaryotic organisms by the physical separation of functions inside specialized organelles.

3. Metabolic pathways are also regulated by other mechanisms that are not related to the architectural design of cells.

Allosteric Modulation

1. Activity of an enzyme can be inhibited or accelerated when small molecules bind to allosteric sites and cause conformational changes in the enzyme.

2. End products may act as allosteric inhibitors by a simple or multiple feedback mechanism on the first enzyme of the pathway.

Covalent Modification

1. Activity of enzymes can be altered by the formation of covalent bonds with modifying groups.

2. The addition of a phosphate group may alter enzyme activity rate.

Regulated and Constitutive Enzymes

1. Inducible enzymes are synthesized only in the presence of substrates.

2. Repressible enzymes are synthesized when products are either absent or present in low concentrations.

3. Constitutive enzymes are always found in the cytoplasm.

Catabolite Repression

1. Some inducible enzymes are not produced if glucose is available as an energy source.

2. Metabolism of glucose reduces the amount of cyclic AMP required for enzyme induction.

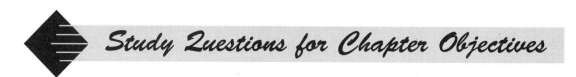

Study Questions for Chapter Objectives

Match the letters in column B to an item in column A. More than one letter from column B may be used.

Column A

____1. Energy-generating reactions
____2. Energy-requiring reactions
____3. Total biochemical reactions in a cell
____4. Light is the source of energy
____5. Chemicals are degraded to release energy
____6. ADP and phosphate form ATP
____7. ATP molecules are converted to ADP and phosphate
____8. Protein molecules are synthesized
____9. Glucose is degraded to O_2, H_2O, and energy
___10. Synthesis of DNA and RNA molecules

Column B

a. Photosynthesis
b. Anabolism
c. Metabolism
d. Catabolism

Quantitative Relationships

Answer *a* if *a* is larger or of greater magnitude than *b*.
Answer *b* if *b* is larger or of greater magnitude than *a*.
Answer c if both are about the same or if neither applies.

___11. More net ATP molecules are produced in:
a. Glycolysis
b. Electron transport

___12. More net ATP molecules are produced in:
a. Glycolysis
b. Citric acid cycle

___13. More reduced NAD molecules are produced in:
a. Glycolysis
b. Citric acid cycle

___14. More ATP molecules are generated in the electron transport chain by:
a. NADH
b. FADH

___15. More ATP molecules are produced by:
a. Fermentation of glucose
b. Aerobic respiration of glucose

___16. More ATP molecules are produced by:
a. Alcoholic fermentation of glucose by yeast
b. Lactic acid fermentation of glucose by lactobacilli

___17. More NADH molecules are produced by:
a. Fermentation of glucose
b. Aerobic respiration of glucose

___18. More energy is needed to activate a chemical reaction in the:
a. Presence of an enzyme
b. Absence of an enzyme

___19. The rate of enzyme action is greater if the environment has:
a. Optimal pH of 7
b. pH of 4

___20. Noncompetitive inhibition of enzyme action is more effective on:
a. Allosteric enzymes
b. Nonallosteric enzymes

Match a letter in column B with an item in column A.

Column A

___21. Lactic acid dehydrogenase
___22. DNA ligase
___23. Cellulase
___24. Phenylalanine deaminase
___25. Phosphorylase
___26. Phosphoglucoisomerase
___27. Transfers electrons and hydrogens
___28. Removes or adds a phosphate group
___29. Rearranges atoms in a molecule
___30. Catalyzes reduction-oxidation reactions

Column B

a. Lyase
b. Isomerase
c. Transferase
d. Oxidoreductase
e. Ligase
f. Hydrolase

31. Describe two roles of ATP in metabolism.

_____

_____

_____

Name the pathways described below.

  a. Electron transport chain
  b. Citric acid cycle
  c. Photosynthesis
  d. Calvin-Benson cycle
  e. Glycolysis

___32. The condensation of acetyl-CoA with oxaloacetic acid begins and ends the pathway.

___33. Glucose is converted to two molecules of pyruvic acid, two molecules of ATP, and two molecules of NADH in the pathway.

___34. Electrons and hydrogens are carried to oxygen by FMN, CoQ, and cytochromes to form H_2O and ATP in the pathway.

___35. Carbon dioxide reacts with ribulose 1, 5-diphosphate to form two molecules of 3-phosphoglycerate, and in six repeats of the pathway, one hexose molecule is formed.

___36. Chlorophyll a molecules absorb light energy and release an electron, which eventually results in the generation of ATP in this pathway.

37. List the final electron acceptor molecules that bacteria use in aerobic and anaerobic respiration.

Aerobic Respiration   **Anaerobic Respiration**

_____   _____

                                           _____

                                           _____

Identify the type of phosphorylation reaction that results in the production of ATP in the following:

38. Glycolysis: _____

39. Electron transport chain: _____

40. Photosynthesis: _____

Fill in the table to identify four mechanisms that control microbial metabolism.

Name of Mechanism	Enzyme Type	How Mechanism Works
Allosteric modulation	Allosteric enzyme	41.
Covalent modification	42.	Enzyme action is increased or slowed if a chemical group is added.
Inducible Enzymes	Genetically-regulated enzyme	43.
Catabolite repression	Inducible enzymes	44.

In the intermediate reactions of glycolysis outlined below, write ATP–>ADP + Pi over the reaction arrow when ATP is required, and write ADP + Pi —> ATP over the reaction arrow when ATP is produced. Count how many ATP molecules are produced and how many are converted to ADP. What is the net number of ATP molecules in this pathway?

45._____

Glucose 46. ————————————> Glucose 6-phosphate 47. ————————————>

Fructose 6-phosphate 48.——————————> Fructose 1,6-diphosphate 49. ——————————>

Glyceraldehyde-3-phosphate and Dihydroxyacetone phosphate 50. ——————————>

Glyceraldehyde-3-phosphate 51. ——————————> 1,3-Diphosphoglycerate 52. ——————————>

3-Phosphoglycerate 53. ——————————> 2-Phosphoglycerate 54. ——————————>

Phosphoenol pyruvate 55. ——————————> Pyruvate

56. In the glycolysis reactions outlined in questions 46 - 55, write NAD + 2H+ —> NADH + H+ over the correct reaction arrow.

57. Explain how NADH will be converted to NAD in fermentation.

_____

_____

58. Explain how NADH will be converted to NAD in aerobic respiration.

_____

_____

For additional practice, write the reactions of the citric acid cycle in sequence. Then write ADP + Pi —> ATP over the correct reaction arrows, and NAD + 2H$^+$ —> NADH + H$^+$ over the correct reaction arrows, and FAD + 2H$^+$ —> FADH + H$^+$ over the correct reaction arrows. Make a tally of the ATP molecules that are produced by substrate phosphorylation. Explain how the reduced NAD and reduced FAD molecules will become oxidized. Explain how the NADH and FADH molecules are related to the production of 34 ATP molecules. See Figure 6-14 in the textbook to guide your answers.

Microbial Genetics

Learning Objectives

1. Differentiate between genotype and phenotype.
2. Describe the process of replication.
3. Differentiate between transcription and translation.
4. Differentiate between an auxotroph and a prototroph.
5. Describe three methods of genetic transfer in procaryotes.
6. Discuss the role of transposons in genetic expression.
7. Describe one mechanism each for repression and induction.
8. Describe the basis of recombinant DNA technology.

Study Outline

Introduction

1. In the middle of the nineteenth century, Gregor Mendel identified discrete structural units responsible for heredity.
2. In 1944, it was demonstrated that genes consist of molecules of DNA.
3. In 1953, James Watson and Sir Francis Crick provided a foundation for molecular genetics by defining the structure of DNA.
4. The major function of genes is to direct the synthesis of proteins and RNA.

Genotype vs. Phenotype

1. The genotype is the sum total of the genetic information contained in an organism.
2. Alterations in genotype occur as a result of mutation or genetic transfer.
3. The phenotype is the sum total of the observable characteristics of an organism.

4. Variations in phenotype are dependent on environmental conditions, such as temperature, available nutrients, and physical state of a culture medium.

Replication and Expression of DNA

1. DNA consists of two chains of complementary nucleotides that form a double helix; DNA is duplicated in a process called replication.
2. Expression of the information contained in DNA involves the production of RNA molecules by a process called transcription.

Replication

1. Replication begins when a helicase enzyme unwinds and separates the two strands of DNA to form a replication fork.
2. In the initial step of replication, a short primer RNA strand is formed on each strand of DNA.

3. Another enzyme binds to the primer RNA and attaches deoxyribonucleotides that are complementary to the parent strand of DNA.

4. The primer RNA is removed by a different enzyme that replaces the ribonucleotides with deoxyribonucleotides.

5. The process of replication is called semiconservative because each of the completed molecules of DNA contains one strand from the parent molecule.

Transcription

1. The base sequence in DNA is the template for the synthesis of the three types of RNA molecules.

2. The strand of DNA that acts as the template for transcription is called the sense strand.

Translation

1. Translation is the process for synthesizing polypeptide chains, or proteins, from the sequence of nitrogen bases on mRNA.

2. The ribosome is the cell structure on which mRNA and activated-tRNA molecules interact for translation.

3. Three nitrogen bases in sequence on mRNA form a codon, and each activated-tRNA has an anticodon, a three base unit, that binds to its complementary codon.

4. The amino acids carried by the tRNA molecules are linked to each other in sequence at the ribosome.

5. The stop codon at the end of the mRNA molecule ends translation, and the polypeptide is released into the cytoplasm.

Mutations

1. Spontaneous mutations rarely affect more than one cell in 10^6 to 10^8 cells.

2. Exposure to some mutagens may cause mutations that affect about one cell in 10^3 cells.

The Parameters of Mutation

1. Mutation is a random and unpredictable event.

2. The mutation rate is the probability that a particular mutation will occur; it is expressed as the average number of mutations per cell per generation.

Types of Mutations

1. Any characteristic of an organism can be altered by a spontaneous or induced mutation.

2. Nutritional mutants are called auxotrophs, and the parent cells from which they are derived are called prototrophs.

3. The most important bacterial mutants in the hospital environment are those that demonstrate resistance to antimicrobial agents.

The Molecular Basis of Mutation

1. Many procaryotes contain small, circular DNA molecules called plasmids, which replicate independently of their hosts.

2. An alteration in base structure of the DNA molecule may be reflected in the placement of a different amino acid at the same relative position on the protein molecule.

3. Since some amino acids may be specified by more than one codon, some base changes on DNA may not cause a change in the amino acid structure of a protein.

Classification of Mutations

1. Alteration of a single base pair on a DNA molecule constitutes a microlesion.

2. Alteration of a number of base pairs or several genes is called a macrolesion.

Point Mutations

1. A point mutation involves a change in a single base of a nucleotide.

2. The consequence of a mutation can be negligible, harmful, or lethal.

Frameshift Mutations

1. The deletion or insertion of a single base can cause a frameshift mutation that results subsequently in the production of nonfunctional proteins.

2. Small deletions occur spontaneously; the loss of extensive DNA is caused by exposure to chemical mutagenic agents or radiations.

Inversions

1. Inversions involve extended sequences of bases.

2. Nonsense codons are very likely with the inversion of some DNA.

Transposons

1. Insertion sequence elements of DNA, known as transposons, occur in procaryotic and some eucaryotic cells.

2. The moveable sequences called transposons (Tns) can affect the expression of a single gene or a cluster of genes.

Reversions

1. Some mutants undergo a mutation that a reversion back to the "wild" type cells or prototrophic cells.
2. The base sequence reverts back to the original sequence.

Detection of Mutants

1. Mutants cells are difficult to detect because there are so few of them in a population.
2. Special cultural techniques are used for detecting mutant cells.

Enrichment of Mutant Cells

1. Mutants that are resistant to antimicrobial agents or phages can be detected by direct enrichment techniques.
2. Penicillin in minimal broth is valuable in selecting for auxotrophs.

Selection for Mutant Cells

1. Nutritionally-deficient mutants can be separated from mixed populations of cells by replica-plating.
2. The auxotrophic mutant cells will grow only on the plate with the needed growth factor.

Detection of Chemical Mutagens

1. The in vitro Ames test uses a histidine-deficient (his⁻) mutant of *Salmonella typhimurium* to detect chemical mutagens.
2. Mutagenic agents promote reversion of *S. typhimurium* his⁻, causing them to grow on discs that contains mutagens on agar plates.

Genetic Transfer in Procaryotic Cells

1. Procaryotes acquire new genetic material from closely related organisms by trans-formation, transduction, and conjugation.
2. Cells that provide DNA in genetic transfer are called donors, whereas cells in which new DNA is introduced are known as recipients.

Transformation

1. Transformation was first observed in strains of *Streptococcus pneumoniae* in 1928 by Frederick Griffith.
2. In 1944, Oswald Avery, Colin MacLeod, and Maclyn McCarty identified the trans-forming substance as DNA.

Transduction

1. Transduction was first demonstrated in 1951 by Joshua and Esther Lederberg and Norton Zinder in strains of *Salmonella typhimurium.*
2. The agents of transfer in transduction are bacteriophages known as transducing or defective particles.

Conjugation

1. Conjugation was discovered in mating types of *Escherichia coli* by Joshua Lederberg and Edward Tatum in 1946.
2. Genetic material is transferred in a single direction after cell-to-cell contact.
3. Donor cells contain a plasmid called the fertility factor; these cells are called F^+ strains.
4. Recipient cells lack the fertility factor and are called F^- strains; after receiving F DNA, they are called F^+ donors.

Regulation of Gene Expression in Procaryotes

1. Inducible enzymes are synthesized only in the presence of substrates.
2. A regulatory gene synthesizes a protein repressor or activator.
3. Operons are genetic units on the bacterial chromosome that control one property; they are regulated by proteins.

Recombination in Eucaryotes

1. Recombination occurs in sexually-reproducing eucaryotes during formation of gametes, and when gametes fuse to form a diploid cell.
2. Pairing of identical chromosomes permits crossing over among the pairs to form new linkage associations of genes.

Recombinant DNA Technology

1. The ability to program cells genetically to perform specific tasks is known as recombinant DNA technology, or genetic engineering.
2. DNA from bacteria, plants, animals, or plasmids can be introduced into host cells to produce recombinant cells.
3. Biomedical, industrial, and agricultural products may be produced using recombinant DNA technology.

Gene Cloning Systems

1. DNA from procaryotic or eucaryotic cells can be transferred to hosts by plasmids, phages, or cosmids.
2. Recombinant cells are cultivated to increase the number of cells tht have copies of the recombined gene of interest.

Selection of Recombinant DNA Hosts

1. Recombinant DNA may be introduced by transformation, transduction, or protoplast fusion.
2. Additional techniques may be used to promote gene expression in the new host cell.
3. Clones may be detected by finding new products, or by nucleic acid hybridization.
4. Nucleic acid hybridization with a DNA or RNA probe can be used to detect recombinant DNA if a product is not expressed.

Gene Amplification

1. Rapid replication of a gene by a polymerase chain reaction (PCR) is called gene amplification.
2. Gene amplification is used to produce high yields of DNA molecules for making biomedical and industrial products, to test for DNA fingerprints, and to test for paternity.

The Ethics of Biochemical Engineering

1. Opponents contend that misuse of information by employers or other agencies may bar applicants from jobs.
2. The possible applications of the mapping of the human genome are of concern to society because of the ethical implications.

Study Questions for Chapter Objectives

Terminology Crossword Puzzle

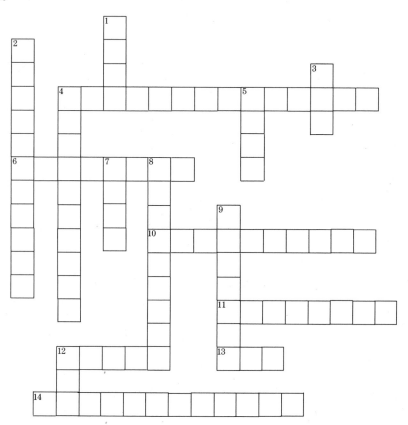

DOWN

1. Acid molecule of ribosome
2. Pilus allows cell mating
3. Amino acid reversion in Ames test
4. DNA segment exits and enters at different places on chromosome
5. Produced by transcription
7. Carrier of amino acids to ribosome
8. All expressed genes that are measured or visualized
9. Circular, closed DNA
12. Method for accumulating millions of DNA copies

ACROSS

4. Naked DNA taken up by a cell that expresses the genes
6. All genes in a cell
10. Building unit for RNA or DNA
11. Change in the base sequence of a gene
12. Small DNA or RNA unit used to detect location of a gene
13. Molecule of heredity
14. When a virus carries bacterial genes to a cell

___1. Gregor Mendel discovered that inheritance in peas occurs in units that are now called:
a. DNA
b. Genotype
c. Genes
d. RNA
e. Plasmids

___2. The structure of DNA was correctly described in 1953 by:
a. Avery, MacLeod, and McCarty
b. Fred Griffith
c. Lederberg
d. Watson and Crick
e. Mendel

___3. The complementary strand of DNA to the following DNA sequence–
A-A-T-T-C-G-T-C-C-A-G-G-T-T-T–is:
a. A-A-T-T-G-C-T-C-C-A-G-G-T-T-T
b. U-U-A-A-G-C-A-G-G-U-C-C-A-A-A
c. T-T-T-T-G-C-T-G-G-T-C-C-T-T-T
d. T-T-A-A-G-C-A-G-G-T-C-C-A-A-A
e. A-A-U-U-G-C-U-G-G-A-C-C-U-U-U

___4. The mRNA strand complementary to the DNA sequence given in question three is:
a. A-A-T-T-G-C-T-C-C-A-G-G-T-T-T
b. U-U-A-A-G-C-A-G-G-U-C-C-A-A-A
c. T-T-T-T-G-C-T-G-G-T-C-C-T-T-T
d. T-T-A-A-G-C-A-G-G-T-C-C-A-A-A
e. A-A-U-U-G-C-U-G-G-A-C-C-U-U-U

___5. The type of mutation that involves the deletion or insertion of one or more bases is:
a. Frameshift
b. Inversion
c. Point
d. Transposons
e. Reversion

___6. Mutations that return the mutant back to its parent type are called:
a. Frameshift
b. Inversion
c. Point
d. Transposons
e. Reversion

___7. Mutants that require more nutrients from their environment in order to grow compared to the parent type cells are called:
a. Auxotrophic
b. Prototrophic
c. "Wild-type"
d. Revertants
e. Recombinant

___8. The microorganisms from which mutants are produced are called:
a. Auxotrophic
b. Prototrophic
c. "Wild-type"
d. Revertants
e. Recombinant

___9. The microorganisms from which auxotrophic mutants are obtained are called:
a. Auxotrophic
b. Prototrophic
c. "Wild-type"
d. Revertants
e. Recombinant

___10. Mutants with a mutation that reverses their mutation are called:
a. Auxotrophic
b. Prototrophic
c. "Wild-type"
d. Revertants
e. Recombinant

Match the items in column A with an item from column B:

Column A

___11. Naked DNA enters a bacterium that expresses genes on the DNA.
___12. The cell must be "competent" for DNA to enter.
___13. Cells must make contact with a like cell by a pilus.
___14. A donor cell provides DNA for a recipient cell.
___15. Plasmid DNA is donated by a cell.
___16. Plasmid DNA is donated by a virus.
___17. Bacterial DNA is carried in a phage.
___18. The recipient cell is a recombinant.
___19. This process was discovered by Fred Griffith.
___20. Hfr cells donate to F⁻ cells.

Column B

a. Transformation
b. Conjugation
c. Transduction
d. Both a and b choices
e. All of a, b, and c choices

Fill in the table by writing in the word or words in the numbered spaces.

Characteristic	Replication	Transcription	Translation
Molecule produced	21.	mRNA	22.
Cell location in procaryote	23.	24.	Ribosome
Cell location in eucaryote	Nucleus	25.	26.
Nucleotides involved	A,C,G,T	27.	28.
Molecular unit that is the building block	29.	Ribonucleotide	30.

31. Describe one mechanism each for repression and induction.

_____

_____

_____

_____

32. Describe the basis of recombinant DNA technology.

_____

_____

_____

33. Describe the role of transposons in genetic expression.

_____

_____

_____

Fill in the blanks at 34, 35, 36, and 37.

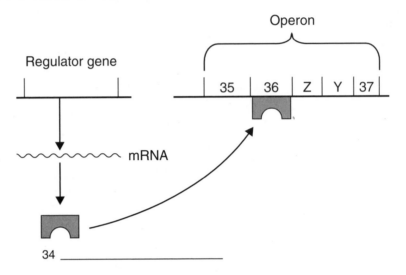

38. What happens when 34 binds to 36? _____

39. What happens when 34 is bound to lactose and cannot bind at 36?_____

_____

MAJOR GROUPS OF MICROORGANISMS

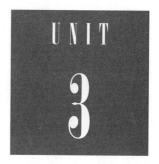

UNIT 3

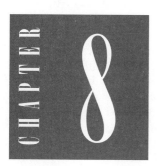

CHAPTER 8

Procaryotes: Bacteria and Archaea

Learning Objectives

1. Explain the concept of species.
2. Describe the derivation of genus and species names.
3. List the major criteria used to classify bacteria and archaea.
4. Explain the significance of chemotaxonomy, nucleic acid relatedness, and genetic recombination in phylogeny of the procaryotes.
5. Name the four divisions to which bacteria and archaea belong.
6. Explain why no classification scheme for procaryotes can be considered complete.

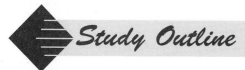

Study Outline

The Concept of Species

1. A bacterial species consists of bacteria that share a large number of characteristics.
2. A newly-discovered bacterium is known as a prototype; a bacterium that differs only slightly is a strain.

How Genus and Species Are Named

1. The binomial system of nomenclature provides a genus and a species name for each bacterium.
2. The authoritative reference for classification of bacteria is *Bergey's Manual of Systematic Bacteriology*.

Ranking the Bacteria

1. Bacteria may be placed in taxons based on similar characteristics or evolutionary relationships.
2. Classification schemes based on phenotype are artificial, but useful.
3. Classification of procaryotes is based on phylogenetic relationships, and it is limited by lack of fossil records and incomplete information.

Criteria for Classifying Bacteria

1. The Gram stain results, growth characteristics, and enzymatic activities aid in the identification of bacteria.

2. Phylogenetic relationships can be detected by serologic, biochemical, and genetic analyses.

Chemotaxonomy

1. Chemotaxonomy uses chemical composition of whole cells or parts of cells to classify bacteria.
2. The chemical nature of cell structures and molecules are analyzed.

Cell Wall Composition

1. Amino acid and carbohydrate composition of peptidoglycan vary among the gram-positive bacteria, but the amino acid composition is nearly the same among gram-negative bacteria.
2. Methods for determining cell wall chemistry are too complex for routine screening.

Plasma Membrane Components

1. The fatty acid content of most bacterial lipids is influenced by the environment, with the exception of the mycolic acids of *Mycobacterium* and *Nocardia.*
2. Phospholipids, glycolipids, and carotenoid composition have significance in taxonomy.

Cytochrome Variables

1. Bacteria contain cytochromes a, b, c, or d; lactic acid bacteria contain only cytochrome b; clostridia have no cytochromes.
2. The study of cytochrome variables requires standard growth conditions.

Amino Acid Sequences

1. Amino acid sequences of proteins, such as ferredoxin, have taxonomic importance.
2. Closely-related bacteria share many amino acid sequences in proteins with the same function.

Protein Profiles

1. Electrophoretically-separated bands of proteins are called fingerprints of bacteria; molecular weights can be assigned to proteins with this method.
2. Such protein profiles are used in the study of epidemics.

Nucleic Acid Relatedness

1. Nucleic acid content is a reliable indicator of relatedness.
2. Nitrogen bases are less subject to frequent change.

DNA Base Composition

1. Mole percent ratios of guanine (G) + cytosine (C) for bacteria range from 25 to 75.

2. Organisms with similar ranges of percent G + C may not be related.

Nucleic Acid Hybridization

1. Degree of relatedness between two organisms can be determined by the degree that DNA strands from the two organisms form hybrid double strands.
2. Double-stranded sequences or duplexes indicate relatedness.

Nucleic Acid Sequences

1. DNA and RNA base sequence studies are powerful techniques for measuring relatedness between two organisms.
2. Sequences of bases in rRNA from the 5S and 16S subunits are different between the bacteria and the archaea, suggesting separate lines of descent for the two types of bacteria.

Genetic Recombination

1. Gene transfer studies are used to establish evolutionary relationships.
2. Plasmids, transposons, and phages contribute to bacterial phenotypic diversity.
3. Lysogeny with particular phages is responsible for toxin production in *Corynebacterium diphtheriae, Streptococcus pyogenes,* and *Clostridium botulinum.*

Numerical Taxonomy

1. Numerical taxonomy relies on a large number of characteristics that are analyzed for similarity in the pattern of results to a known prototype organism by specialized computer software bacteria.
2. The operational taxonomic units (OTUs) can be genera, species, or strains.
3. Only 10 to 20 percent of total genetic potential is revealed by numerical taxonomy.

The Bacteria

1. All bacteria belong to the divisions Gracilicutes, Firmicutes, or Tenericutes.
2. *Bergey's Manual of Systematic Bacteriology* contains 33 sections that describe the groups of bacteria; the groups exemplify the diversity of morphology, biochemical activities, and habitats.

The Spirochetes

1. Spirochetes are helically shaped, motile organisms that live in water or in human or animal hosts.
2. Examples of pathogenic spirochetes are *Treponema pallidum* (syphilis), *Borrelia burgdorferi* (Lyme disease), and *Leptospira interrogans* (a human and animal pathogen).

Aerobic/Microaerophilic Helical Vibrioid Gram-Negative Bacteria

1. The motile vibrioids live in fresh or coastal waters; some cause disease; some are bacterial or algal predators.
2. The microaerophilic species of *Campylobacter* have special atmospheric requirements.

Gram-Negative Aerobic Rods and Cocci

1. These bacteria are widely distributed in nature; many are pathogens, such as *Neisseria gonorrhoeae* (gonorrhea) and *Bordetella pertussis* (whooping cough).
2. *Rhizobium* species fix atmospheric nitrogen when growing in root nodules of leguminous plants such as soybeans and clover.

Facultatively Anaerobic Gram-Negative Rods

1. Members of this large group are found in soil, water, and in the intestinal tracts of animals and humans.
2. *Escherichia coli* is the best known enteric organism.

Anaerobic Gram-Negative Rods

1. These bacteria are either straight, curved, or helical; motile or nonmotile; and they are found in the intestinal tract and in dental plaque.
2. *Bacteroides,* a resident of the human intestinal tract, causes anaerobic bacteremia, rectal abscesses, and other infections.

Anaerobic Gram-Negative Cocci

1. These bacteria are found in the mouth, intestine, and vagina.
2. Their role in disease is uncertain.

The Rickettsias and Chlamydias

1. Rickettsias and chlamydias are gram-negative rods or cocci that multiply in host cells and not on artificial cultivation media.
2. Chlamydias cause trachoma and at least two sexually transmitted diseases in humans.

Mycoplasmas

1. Mycoplasmas have no cell wall; they are the smallest of the free-living bacteria.
2. Mycoplasmas cause disease in animals, plants, and humans.

Gram-Positive Cocci

1. These bacteria are aerobic or anaerobic; some may be harmless, and others are pathogenic.

2. *Staphylococcus aureus, Streptococcus pneumoniae,* and *Streptococcus pyogenes* are important human pathogens.
3. Species of *Peptococcus* and *Peptostreptococcus* cause anaerobic infections.

Endospore-Forming Gram-Positive Rods and Cocci

1. The spores of the gram-positive rods and cocci are resistant to heat and disinfectants.
2. Species of *Bacillus* and *Clostridium* are important in the food industry and in medicine.

Regular Nonsporing Gram-Positive Rods

1. These bacteria have complex nutritional requirements.
2. Some lactobacilli are found in the mouth, intestinal tract, and vagina; other lactobacilli are responsible for fermented foods and beverages.
3. *Listeria monocytogenes* causes an inflammatory disease of the brain and meninges.

Irregular Nonsporing Gram-Positive Rods

1. These bacteria have unusual shapes that are clublike and pleomorphic, and they are either facultatively anaerobic or obligately aerobic.
2. The most important pathogen of the group is *Corynebacterium diphtheriae.*

Mycobacteria

1. These bacteria are aerobic acid-fast rods that form filaments; the high lipid content of their cell walls is responsible for the acid-fast staining characteristic.
2. *Mycobacterium tuberculosis* and *M. leprae* are the most important pathogens of the group.

Nocardioforms

1. These bacteria are aerobic, gram-positive, and produce hyphae.
2. Species of *Nocardia* grow on laboratory cultivation media; they can cause infection in the human lungs or skin.

Streptomycetes and Their Allies

1. These bacteria have a soil habitat; they resemble the filamentous *Actinomyces,* but they are aerobic.
2. *Streptomyces* are important for the production of antibiotics.

The Archaea

1. Archaea live in unusual or extreme habitats such as hot acid springs, extremely saline environments, and anaerobic soils.

2. The lack of peptidoglycan in the cell walls of most archaea, except for the thermoacidophiles, is a distinctive characteristic. Archaea are members of the division Mendosicutes.

3. The chemistry of lipids and rRNA molecules are different from most other cell types; they distinguish archaea from eucaryotes and bacteria.

The Methanogens

1. The methanogens grow in anaerobic environments such as swamps and marshes; all members produce methane.

2. Some methanogens are endosymbionts in anaerobic protozoa.

The Extreme Thermophiles

1. The extreme thermophiles can grow at temperatures up to 150°C under high hydrostatic pressure in deep ocean springs.

2. Many grow in highly-acidic environments such as the Yellowstone hot springs.

The Extreme Halophiles

1. The extreme halophiles are found in salt lakes, salt-evaporating ponds, and in brines that have salt concentrations from 9 to 32 percent.

2. No foodborne illnesses have been described due to the presence of these organisms in brines used for food preservation.

 Study Questions for Chapter Objectives

Write the names of the four divisions under which bacteria are classified. Write the type of bacteria (either gram-negative or gram-positive) and one or two other characteristics of the division.

Division Name

1. _____

3. _____

5. _____

7. _____

Bacteria Type

2. _____

4. _____

6. _____

8. _____

Match a letter in column B with an item in column A to describe the concept of species.

Column A

____9. Interbreeding determines the species.

____10. Asexual reproduction is the primary means of population growth.

____11. Many stable characteristics over many generations

____12. Offspring may mutate independently of parent cells by gene transfers and selective environmental pressures.

Column B

a. Bacteria
b. Plants and animals

13. The system of using two names to identify an organism is called:

_____

_____

Circle the correct word.

14. The genus is the (first/second) name.

15. The first letter of the genus name is always (capitalized/lowercase).

16. The species is the (first/second) name.

17. The first letter of the species name is always (capitalized/lowercase).

Fill in the blank:

Both genus and species names are written or printed by using either:

18. _____ letters or by 19. _____ the name.

20. A prototype is the organism that was first identified, and its characteristics have been described for the species. What is the term for a bacterium that has most, but not all, of the same characteristics, but is still identified as the same species?

_____

List two major criteria used to assign bacteria into one of the four divisions.

21. _____

22. _____

23. If the following results on moles percent G + C were found in three unknown organisms, what conclusion would you reach on relatedness? What other tests on nucleic acids would you recommend for clarification?

Organism	Moles % G + C
A	62-65
B	31-36
C	59-64

_____

_____

_____

Match the organism with the description of its group.

Organism	Group
___24. *Treponema pallidum*	a. Mycoplasmas
___25. *Campylobacter* sp.	b. Spirochetes
___26. *Bacillus anthracis*	c. Gram-positive cocci
___27. *Neisseria gonorrhoeae*	d. Endospore-forming
___28. *Spiroplasma citri*	e. Acid-fast
___29. *Staphylococcus aureus*	f. Snapping division
___30. *Corynebacterium diphtheriae*	g. Facultatively anaerobic
___31. *Mycobacterium tuberculosis*	h. Microaerophilic vibrioid
___32. *Escherichia coli*	i. Microaerophilic gram-negative cocci
___33. *Veillonella* sp.	j. Anaerobic gram-negative cocci

34. What characteristics of archaea make them different from eucaryotes and bacteria?

_____

_____

_____

_____

_____

35. Explain why no classification scheme for procaryotes can be considered complete.

_____

_____

_____

_____

_____

_____

_____

Match a letter in column B with an item in column A.

Column A	Column B
___36. Analyzes the chemical nature of cell structures and molecules.	a. Numerical taxonomy
___37. Analyzes the degree of binding between two strands of DNA from two bacteria.	b. DNA base sequence c. DNA hybridization d. Percent G + C
___38. Analyzes the order of bases on the DNA strand.	e. Chemotaxonomy
___39. Analyzes 50 or more characteristics for similarity by computer analyses.	
___40. Analyzes the percentage of guanine and cytosine, relative to all four bases in the DNA molecule.	

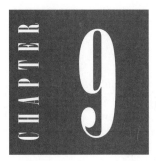

CHAPTER 9

Eucaryotes: Algae, Protozoa, and Fungi

Learning Objectives

1. Describe the major characteristics of algae, protozoa, and fungi.
2. Explain what advantage colonization has for algae.
3. Describe the basis used for classifying algae into the major divisions.
4. Describe the basis for classifying fungi.
5. Differentiate between acellular and cellular slime molds.

Study Outline

Algae

1. Algae are microscopic or macroscopic organisms that contain chlorophylls and accessory pigments called phycobilins.
2. Motile algae have one or more flagella.
3. Algae reproduce asexually; sexual reproduction occurs by the formation of sex cells, the gametes.

Ranking the Algae

1. Algae do not have true roots, stems, and leaves.
2. The types of photopigments, cell wall chemistry, the type of reproduction, and the types of reserve materials are important in classifying algae.

Green Algae (Chlorophyta)

1. Green algae contain chlorophylls *a* and *b,* and carotenes, and the cell wall contains cellulose and pectin.
2. *Chlamydomonas* and *Chlorella* are unicellular; *Volvox* and *Spirogyra* are examples of multicellular green algae.

Euglenoids (Euglenophyta)

1. Euglenoids are unicellular; they contain chlorophylls *a* and *b,* carotenes, two anterior flagella, and no cell wall. The outer layer is a flexible pellicle.
2. A stigma (red eyespot) directs euglenoids toward the light.

Diatoms, Yellow-Green, and Golden-Brown Algae (Chrysophyta)

1. An abundance of carotenes is responsible for the golden–brown coloring of some members of the division.
2. Diatoms have two-part cell walls containing silica that form intricate patterns.
3. Reproduction by mitosis produces smaller diatoms at each division; sexual reproduction restores the small diatoms to their original size.

Brown Algae (Phaeophyta)

1. Brown algae are large, complex multicellular organisms resembling plants; the color of brown algae is due to fucoxanthin pigment.

2. Brown algae are marine kelp; rootlike holdfasts anchor the kelp on rocks and other surfaces in the ocean.

3. Algin, a component of algal cell walls, is a commercially useful product.

Dinoflagellates (Pyrrophyta)

1. Dinoflagellates are primarily unicellular marine algae; they contain a variety of pigments; some emit light.

2. Their two-plate cell walls contain cellulose and silica; most species reproduce by longitudinal binary fission.

Red Algae (Rhodophyta)

1. Red algae live in surface waters or in depths of up to 100 meters or more; their color is due to phycoerythrin.

2. Agar is obtained from species of *Gelidium* and *Gracilaria;* it is commercially important, especially for microbiological culture media.

Protozoa

1. Protozoa are unicellular organisms that contain no cell walls or photopigments.

2. The feeding stages of protozoa are called trophozoites; nonfeeding thick-walled resistant stages are called cysts.

3. A small number of protozoa cause human disease.

Ranking the Protozoa

1. Protozoa are classified according to the mode of motility and cell structure; some protozoa are nonmotile as adults.

2. Euglenoids and dinoflagellates have characteristics of both algae and protozoa.

Pseudopods (Sarcodina)

1. Amebas move by false feet called pseudopodia.

2. Six species of parasitic amebas and a few free-living species cause human disease.

3. *Entamoeba histolytica* causes amoebic dysentery.

Flagellates (Mastigophora)

1. Flagellates have one or more anterior flagella.

2. Intestinal protozoa remain in place because sucking discs protect them from peristaltic action.

3. *Giardia lamblia, Trichomonas vaginalis,* and the trypanosomes of African sleeping sickness cause human disease.

Ciliates (Ciliata)

1. Ciliates have short, hairlike appendages called cilia, that extend from their plasma membranes.

2. They have at least one macronucleus, and one or more micronucleii.

3. *Balantidium coli* is the only ciliate known to cause human disease.

Sporozoans (Sporozoa)

1. The malarian parasites, belonging to the genus *Plasmodium,* have complex life cycles that require vertebrate hosts and mosquitoes.

2. All members of the class are parasites in one or more hosts.

Fungi

1. The fungi are a large, diverse group that includes unicellular yeasts, multicellular molds, mushrooms, and other organisms.

2. Dimorphic fungi have either a yeast or mold stage of growth, depending on environmental conditions.

3. The basic structure of mold growth is the formation of tubular filaments called hyphae, either with separations between cells (septa), which make the hyphae septate, or no separations, which make them nonseptate hyphae.

4. A mass of intertwined hyphae makes up a mycelium.

5. All fungi lack photopigments, and most have cell walls of chitin.

6. Fungi are major decomposers of dead organic matter, but some are attracted to living tissue.

Ranking the Fungi

1. Fungi are classified according to their type of hyphae, mode of reproduction, and type of reproductive spores.

2. The five types of asexual spores are 1) arthrospores, 2) blastospores, 3) chlamydospores, 4) conidiospores, and 5) sporangiospores.

3. Sexual spores are produced if two organisms of opposite mating type are cultivated together.

Water Molds (Zygomycota)

1. Water molds have nonseptate hyphae and produce sporangiospores.

2. Zygospores are produced when hyphae of different mating strains fuse.

Sac Fungi (Ascomycota)

1. The sac fungi consist of yeasts and some molds with septate hyphae.

2. Blastospores or microconidia are produced asexually; ascospores are sexual spores.

3. Some yeasts are used to make bread, beer, and wine.

4. Several plant diseases are caused by molds of this class.

Club Fungi (Basidiomycota)

1. Rusts, smuts, mushrooms, and toadstools are club fungi.

2. The fungi produce clublike basidia from which develop the sexual spores, or basidiospores.

3. The mushroom *Amanita phalloides* produces dangerous hallucinogenic toxins.

4. *Cryptococcus neoformans* causes pulmonary disease and meningitis in humans.

Imperfect Fungi (Deuteromycota)

1. The imperfect fungi are not known to reproduce sexually.

2. Many of the imperfect fungi are dimorphic; some produce more than one type of asexual spore.

3. Some members cause superficial infections of the skin and some systemic mycoses.

Slime Molds

1. Slime molds have properties of both the protozoa and fungi.

2. They produce fruiting bodies at one stage in their life cycles.

Acellular Slime Molds

1. Acellular slime molds are masses of cytoplasm with many nuclei called a plasmodium.

2. Fruiting bodies appear when growth stops.

3. Spores released from fruiting bodies germinate, fuse, and form a new plasmodium.

Cellular Slime Molds

1. Cellular slime molds resemble amebas.

2. The cells form a pseudoplasmodium if food supplies are inadequate.

3. Fruiting bodies arise from pseudoplasmodia and release spores.

 Study Questions for Chapter Objectives

Match the description of the organism in column A with an organism in column B. An organism may be selected more than once.

Column A	Column B
___1. Filamentous alga	a. *Gelidium*
___2. Movement by pseudopodia	b. *Balantidium*
___3. Production of toxin	c. *Paramecium*
___4. Presence of phycoerythrin	d. *Aspergillus*
___5. Spherical colonies	e. *Spirogyra*
___6. Movement by cilia	f. *Giardia*
___7. Single chloroplast	g. *Claviceps*
___8. Movement by flagella	h. *Entamoeba*
___9. No sexual spores	i. *Volvox*
__10. Source of agar	j. *Chlamydomonas*

Match the letters from column B with each item in column A. More than one letter may be used from column B.

Column A

___11. Unicellular
___12. Multicellular
___13. Photopigments present
___14. Cell walls present
___15. Structures for motility present
___16. Pseudopodia
___17. Protista
___18. Includes *Chlamydomonas* and *Volvox*.
___19. Includes yeasts, molds, mushrooms, smuts, rusts.
___20. Includes *Entamoeba histolytica*

Column B

a. Fungi
b. Algae
c. Protozoa
d. Algae and fungi
e. Algae and protozoa
f. Fungi and protozoa

Write three criteria for classifying algae into different divisions.

21. _____

22. _____

23. _____

Fill in the table at number 24 to 29 below with the appropriate words for separating protozoa into classes.

Class Name	Mode of Motility	Reproduction Type
Sarcodina	24.	Binary fission
25.	Flagella	26.
Sporozoa	27.	Multiple fission
Ciliata	28.	29.

Match a letter from column B with an item in column A. A letter may be used more than once.

Column A

___30. Has a plasmodium.
___31. Has a pseudoplasmodium.
___32. Many nuclei inside a mass of cytoplasm constitute this organism.
___33. Produce fruiting bodies that release spores.
___34. Individual cells migrate within the slug stage.

Column B

a. Acellular slime mold
b. Cellular slime mold
c. True for both types

Match a letter from column B with an item in column A. A letter may be used more than once.

Column A

___35. Zygospores are the sexual spore.
___36. Hypha is nonseptate.
___37. Hypha is septate.
___38. Basidiospores are formed sexually.
___39. Sexual spore formation is unknown.
___40. Ascospores are formed sexually.
___41. Arthroconidia and other conidia are formed asexually.
___42. Asexual conidia are usually absent.
___43. Water molds are included.
___44. Yeast are included.
___45. Mushrooms are included.

Column B

a. Ascomycota
b. Basidiomycota
c. Deuteromycota
d. Zygomycota

46. Differentiate between a trophozoite and a cyst stage in the life cycle of protozoa.

_____

_____

_____

_____

_____

47. Explain an advantage of colonization for algae.

_____

_____

_____

_____

CHAPTER 10 Viruses

Learning Objectives

1. Define capsid, capsomere, virion, nucleocapsid.
2. Explain the basis for classification of viruses into two major groups.
3. Describe three major morphological types of viruses.
4. Describe the sequence of events occurring in the replicative cycle of viruses.
5. List three in vitro methods of cultivating viruses.
6. Explain the significance of the 50 percent infectious dose (ID_{50}).
7. Explain the difference between a lytic cycle and lysogeny.
8. Describe the role of reverse transcriptase in cells infected with retroviruses.

Study Outline

The Structure and Specificity of Viruses

1. The extracellular inert phase of viruses is known as a virion.
2. The protein coat of viruses is called a capsid.
3. The nucleic acid and protein coat are the nucleocapsid.

Shape and Size

1. Most nucleocapsids have helical or polyhedral symmetry.
2. Some nucleocapsids are enclosed in an envelope of host cell membrane or viral origin; some envelopes carry glycoprotein spikes. Nonenveloped viruses are described as naked.
3. Some bacteriophages have heads with icosahedral symmetry and tails attached to end plates.
4. Poxviruses have brick-shaped virions with the nucleic acid arranged as a tubular structure in a crisscross pattern.

Host Range and Specificity

1. Some viruses infect a particular type of cell; others infect many types of cells.
2. Plasma membranes of cells contain receptors that bind to antigens on viruses.

Classification of Viruses

1. Viruses are classified according to the type of nucleic acid in their cores.
2. The molecular weight of nucleic acid strands, the size and shape of virions, nucleocapsid symmetry, and strategy of replication are important distinguishing characteristics.
3. The DNA viruses and double-stranded RNA viruses require transcription to mRNA.
4. Reverse transcriptase is responsible for making a copy of DNA from RNA.
5. Family or group names are used in classifying viruses.

Replication of Viruses

1. Resources of host cells are used for viral replication.
2. The infectious process involves an orderly series of events.

Attachment

1. The initial contact between viruses and susceptible cells is a random collision.
2. The receptors on host cells are often proteins.

Penetration

1. Viruses may or may not participate in viral penetration into cells.
2. Penetration is sometimes made possible by fusion of the plasma membrane and a virus.

Uncoating

1. Uncoating nucleic acids of viruses occurs during or after penetration.
2. Capsids of bacteriophages never enter host cells.
3. Capsids of other virions are destroyed within cells by cellular or viral enzymes.

Multiplication

1. Multiplication of viruses takes place either in the nucleus or the cytoplasm of host cells.
2. Viral nucleic acids supply genetic information for producing more virions.
3. Transcription of RNA from host DNA ceases almost immediately after penetration.

Assembly

1. Assembly sometimes requires viral-coded enzymes.
2. The eclipse period is the period from entry of a virus into a host cell and the appearance of infectious progeny.
3. Eclipse periods range from two to 20 hours.

Release

1. Mature progeny are liberated by cell lysis or budding.
2. Movement of assembled virions promotes incorporation of cellular proteins into viral capsids or envelopes.
3. A bacterium produces 200 or more infective particles; a human cell makes 10^5 to 10^6 infective particles.

Hidden Viruses

1. Some viruses establish stable carrier states in infected cells.
2. Integrated genes of viruses are transcribed or may alter expression of a host's genes.

Lysogeny

1. A phage loses its ability to produce a lytic cycle when viral DNA is integrated into a host bacterium.
2. The integrated phage is called a prophage, and the relationship with the host cell is known as lysogeny.
3. The expression of one or more new characteristics by the bacterium that hosts a prophage is described as lysogenic conversion.
4. The ability of *Corynebacterium diphtheriae, Streptococcus pyogenes,* and *Clostridium botulinum* to produce toxins is the result of lysogenic conversion.
5. A prophage can revert to a lytic phage either spontaneously or in response to an environmental factor.

Latency

1. Some viruses exist as proviruses in a latent stage of eucaryotic cells.
2. Proviruses may be reactivated by host or environmental factors.
3. Latent periods for proviruses are unpredictable.

Cultivation of Viruses

1. Type-specific bacteriophages can be grown by adding phages to a culture of susceptible bacteria.
2. Phage particles can be harvested after lysis of host cells.
3. Animal viruses grow in 1) embryonated eggs, 2) cell cultures, or 3) animals.

Embryonated Eggs

1. The influenza, rabies, canine distemper, and mumps viruses are propagated in embryonated chicken eggs.
2. The required age of the embryo and the specific route of inoculation into the embryonated egg vary according to the virus.
3. Lesions may occur on membranes, or viruses may be present in embryonic fluids.

Cell Cultures

1. Viruses may be grown in primary or continuous host cell lines.
2. Primary cell cultures may be transferred a limited number of times, but continuous cell lines can be transferred an indefinite number of times.

3. A morphological change known as a cytopathic effect (CPE) occurs in some virus-infected cells.

Animals

1. A variety of animals are used for isolation of viruses from clinical specimens of infections or tumors.
2. Viruses can be isolated from nasal or throat washings, urine, or other body fluids.

Enumeration of Viruses

1. A count of physical particles provides limited information.
2. An assay that measures infectivity is more meaningful.

Particle Counts

1. Electron microscopes can be used to count large viruses.
2. The highest dilution of virus causing red blood cells to agglutinate is a method for quantitating some viruses.

Infectivity Assays

1. The highest dilution of virus causing infection of embryonated eggs, cell cultures, or animals is the infectious dose.
2. The titer is expressed as the 50 percent infectious dose, or ID_{50}.
3. The plaque method mixes host cells with susceptible cells and nutrient agar.
4. Each plaque, produced by progeny of a single infectious particle, is a plaque-forming unit (PFU).
5. The efficiency of plating (EOP) is obtained by comparing the ID_{50} with the electron microscope count.

The Major DNA Viruses of Vertebrates

1. All of the DNA viruses contain double-stranded DNA except for the parvoviruses and hepadnaviruses.
2. All have icosahedral symmetry except the poxviruses.

Parvoviruses

1. These are the smallest of the DNA viruses; some parvoviruses depend on a helper virus to initiate infection.
2. Parvoviruses are best known as causes of animal diseases.
3. Parvovirus B19 causes "fifth disease" in children and one type of aplastic anemia.

Hepadnaviruses

1. The most studied hepadnavirus is hepatitis B virus (HBV).
2. The major polypeptide of the HBV is hepatitis B surface antigen (HBsAg), which is used in the HBV vaccine.

Papovaviruses

1. The double-stranded DNA of papovaviruses serves as a template for mRNA and progeny.
2. The papillomaviruses cause benign and malignant warts in humans; they are suspected of causing cervical cancer.

Adenoviruses

1. Only half of the 42 human adenoviruses cause disease.
2. Human adenoviruses cause respiratory, gastrointestinal, genitourinary, and eye infections.

Herpesviruses

1. Herpesviruses contain envelopes acquired by budding from the nuclear and plasma membranes of host cells.
2. All herpesviruses can remain latent for years and cause recurrent disease.
3. Fever blisters, genital herpes, chicken-pox, cytomegalovirus infection, and infectious mononucleosis are caused by herpesviruses.
4. The Epstein-Barr virus (EBV) is associated with Burkitt's lymphoma and naso-pharyngeal cancer in some parts of the world.

Poxviruses

1. Poxviruses are the largest and most complex of the DNA viruses.
2. The virion contains DNA-dependent DNA and RNA polymerases; these are the only DNA viruses that replicate in the cytoplasm.
3. Vaccinia (cowpox) and molluscum contagiosum (a benign tumor in humans) are caused by poxviruses.

The Major RNA Viruses of Vertebrates

1. Most RNA viruses contain single-stranded RNA.
2. The group contains helical or icosahedral nucleocapsid symmetry and may or may not have envelopes.
3. Replication often requires replicative intermediates (RIs) and RNA-DNA hybrids.

4. Multiplication usually occurs in the cytoplasm.

Reoviruses

1. Reoviruses were once called "respiratory enteric orphans."

2. Rotaviruses cause serious disease of children in developing countries; they are also one cause of travelers' diarrhea.

Picornaviruses

1. Picornaviruses are the smallest of the RNA viruses.

2. The single strand of RNA acts directly as mRNA or as a template for a replicative form (RF).

3. Viruses that cause poliomyelitis, coxsackie disease, hepatitis A, some enteric infections, and most common colds are in this group.

Togaviruses

1. Togaviruses are enveloped particles with nucleocapsid symmetry.

2. Many togaviruses are transmitted by arthropod vectors; they may replicate in the vector and animal hosts.

3. Viruses causing rubella, eastern equine encephalitis (EEE), and western equine encephalitis (WEE) belong to this group.

Flaviviruses

1. Flaviviruses resemble togaviruses in structure.

2. They replicate alternately in arthropod vectors and vertebrate hosts.

3. Yellow fever, St. Louis encephalitis, Japanese B encephalitis, and hepatitis C are caused by flaviviruses.

Orthomyxoviruses

1. Orthomyxoviruses are roughly spherical, have envelopes, and demonstrate helical nucleocapsid symmetry.

2. The envelopes contain a hemagglutinin antigen (HA) and a neuraminidase (NA).

3. RNA, complementary to virion RNA, is the template for mRNA, progeny, and an RI.

4. Influenza viruses A, B, and C are orthomyxoviruses.

5. Different strains of influenza viruses A and B occur as a result of phenomena known as antigenic shift and antigenic drift.

Paramyxoviruses

1. Paramyxoviruses are pleomorphic, enveloped viruses with helical nucleocapsid symmetry.

2. Viral antigens are often found on plasma membranes of infected cells.

3. Measles, mumps, and respiratory syncytial viruses are paramyxoviruses.

Rhabdoviruses

1. Rhabdoviruses are bullet-shaped, enveloped, and have helical nucleocapsid symmetry.

2. Rabies is the most serious infection caused by a rhabdovirus.

Bunyaviruses

1. Bunyaviruses, the largest group of mammalian viruses, resemble influenza viruses.

2. Some are transmitted by mosquitoes, sand flies, and ticks; others are spread by aerosolized excreta of rodents.

3. Hemorrhagic fever, kidney dysfunction, and acute respiratory disease are caused by bunyaviruses.

Retroviruses

1. Retroviruses are spherical enveloped virions having helical ribonucleoproteins and icosahedral nucleocapsids.

2. The viruses code for the enzyme reverse transcriptase, which transcribes a DNA molecule from the viral RNA.

3. The DNA copy of retroviral RNA may exist as a provirus in host cells.

4. Some retroviruses cause cancer in animals with oncogenes.

5. The human immunodeficiency virus (HIV) is a retrovirus that causes acquired immunodeficiency syndrome (AIDS); it infects human cells with CD4 receptors.

Lesser Known Viruses

1. Filoviruses and calciviruses cause zoonoses.

2. Animal reservoirs for the filoviruses Marburg and Ebola, which cause hemorrhagic fever, are unknown.

3. Calciviruses cause many animal diseases, but the Norwalk agent causes gastroenteritis in humans.

Viruses and Human Cancer

1. Cancer is a multicausal disease, but it is likely that viruses are involved in some types of cancer.

2. Environmental and host factors are important in establishing the disease.

Viroids, Virusoids, and Prions

1. Disease-associated infectious particles are viroids, virusoids, and prions.
2. Some of the subviral entities increase rapidly under appropriate conditions.

Viroids

1. Viroids range in size from 15 to 100 nm; they cause diseases in some plants.
2. Some consist of single-stranded RNA only with no capsid; others have envelopes that surround the RNA.

Virusoids

1. Virusoids approximate viroids in size and parasitize helper viruses.

2. A larger RNA plant virus provides the genetic information for their replication.

Prions

1. Prions are infectious protein particles that are extremely heat-resistant.
2. Their existence is in question because proteins are not known to replicate.
3. Kuru, Creutzfeld-Jakob disease, scrapie, (a disease of sheep), and bovine spongiform encephalopathy (mad cow disease) are associated with prions.

 Study Questions for Chapter Objectives

Match the disease in column A with the group to which the etiologic agent belongs in column B.

Column A	**Column B**
___ 1. Infectious mononucleosis	a. Orthomyxovirus
___ 2. "Fifth disease"	b. Rhabdovirus
___ 3. Warts	c. Papovavirus
___ 4. Shipyard eye	d. Herpesvirus
___ 5. AIDS	e. Togavirus
___ 6. Polio	f. Parvovirus
___ 7. Measles	g. Adenovirus
___ 8. Rubella	h. Retrovirus
___ 9. Influenza	i. Picornavirus
___ 10. Rabies	j. Paramyxovirus

11. Identify the basis for classification of viruses into two major groups.

_____

_____

_____

Match terms in column A with their definition in column B.

Column A	**Column B**
___ 12. Capsid	a. Association of nucleic acid with protein
___ 13. Capsomere	b. Single inert particle
___ 14. Envelope	c. Single protein unit of protein coat
___ 15. Spike	d. Protein coat
___ 16. Nucleocapsid	e. Host cell membrane layer over capsid
___ 17. Virion	f. Glycoprotein molecule in envelope

List three major morphological types of nucleocapsid symmetry in viruses.

18. _____

19. _____

20. _____

List the six stages in the replication of viruses with a brief description of the stage.
      Stage   **Description**

21. _____

22. _____

23. _____

24. _____

25. _____

26. _____

Next to each bacterial cell in the diagram below, write in the stage of the lytic cycle that the bacteriophage is undergoing.

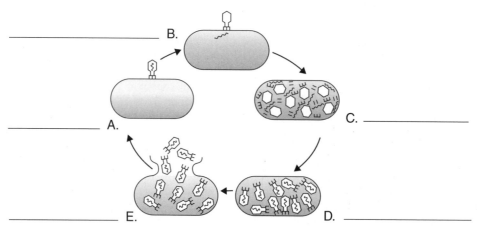

27.   Explain the difference between a lytic cycle of virus replication, and lysogeny.

_____

_____

_____

_____

28. What is meant by lysogenic conversion?

_____

_____

_____

_____

29. List three common methods for cultivating viruses.

_____

_____

_____

_____

30. Explain what is meant by cytopathic effects (CPEs).

_____

_____

_____

31. Explain the significance of ID$_{50}$.

_____

_____

_____

_____

32. Describe the role of reverse transcriptase in retrovirus infections.

_____

_____

_____

_____

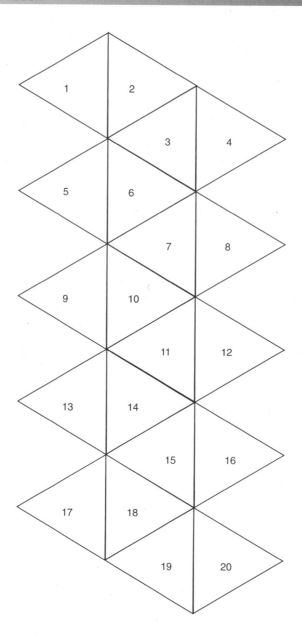

Virus Model Exercise: You will find a numbered diagram above that is the model of a twenty-sided figure that represents the polyhedral shape of a virus capsid.

Necessary materials: Card stock paper, scissors, tape

1. The model will look better and fold easier if you photocopy this page onto a sheet of card-stock paper (similar to paper used in 3"x 5" index cards). This will produce a more sturdy three-dimensional model.

2. Cut out the diagram on the outside lines only.

3. Gently fold the diagram in half between numbers 10 and 11.

4. Continue to gently fold all the lines.

5. Bend the edges of the model together so that triangle 1 meets triangle 17, and triangle 2 meets triangle 19. Tape these edges together.

6. Bend the edges of triangle 4 to meet triangle 20, and tape edges together.

7. Bend the edges of all the other triangles to meet the opposite triangles, and tape the edges together to form a three-dimensional viral capsid model.

HOST-PARASITE RELATIONSHIPS

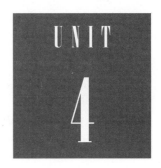

UNIT

4

11 Epidemiology of Infectious Diseases

Learning Objectives

1. Differentiate between an infectious disease and a communicable disease.
2. Define epidemic, pandemic, and endemic.
3. Explain the role of carriers in communicable diseases.
4. Describe three types of epidemiological investigations.
5. Explain how infectious diseases are classified.
6. Differentiate between a reservoir and a mode of transmission.
7. Contrast the role of the Centers for Disease Control and Prevention (CDC) with that of the Occupational Safety and Health Administration (OSHA) in public health.

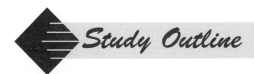

Study Outline

Introduction

1. Epidemiology is the study of the how, when, and where of diseases that occur within populations.
2. John Snow was the first to identify a common source for bacteria causing cholera in London in 1849.
3. Data collected by epidemiologists is useful in prevention and treatment of infectious diseases.

Classifying Community Diseases

1. An epidemic is characterized by an unusually large number of cases in a community within a short period of time.

2. A pandemic exists when an epidemic spreads through many parts of the world.
3. A disease is characterized as being endemic if it is present in a limited number of persons within a geographic area at all times.
4. If a disease occurs without regularity in a community, it is described as sporadic.
5. A carrier harbors an infectious agent in the absence of disease.
6. A transient carrier sheds pathogens for several days or months; a chronic carrier can shed an infectious agent for months or years.
7. Immunity within a population is herd immunity.

Methods of Epidemiology

1. Epidemiologists use three types of investigations: 1) descriptive, 2) analytical, and 3) experimental.
2. Infectious disease practitioners perform surveys in hospitals.

Descriptive Epidemiology

1. Descriptive epidemiology is a retrospective study of a disease.
2. Data is accumulated over a given period of time.

Analytical Epidemiology

1. Analytical epidemiology looks for common characteristics or risk factors to establish a cause-and-effect relationship.
2. Comparisons are made between ill people and a matched group of healthy individuals called cohorts.

Experimental Epidemiology

1. Sometimes a hypothesis can be established and tested if data is analyzed over a time period.
2. Common habits, places of exposure, or sources can often be identified.

Assessments of Disease Frequency

Prevalence and Incidence

1. Prevalence is the total number of cases or percentage of individuals having a disease at a point in time.
2. Incidence is the rate of new cases during a specified time interval compared to the number of healthy people in the population.

Morbidity and Mortality Rates

1. Morbidity (illness) and mortality (death) rates reflect important trends valuable in surveillance.
2. Data is used by public health agencies, other state and federal regulatory agencies, and medical advisory councils to make recommendations to protect public health.

Types of Infectious Diseases

1. The primary classification of infectious diseases is based on etiologic agents.
2. Other classifications provide less specific, but important information.

Primary and Secondary Diseases

1. A primary disease is the initial disease; a disease following primary disease is called a secondary disease.
2. Bacterial infections may follow viral diseases as secondary invaders.

3. Microorganisms causing secondary disease may be a part of the normal flora or have an environmental origin.

Opportunistic Diseases

1. Opportunistic diseases are caused by microorganisms that are usually nonpathogens or pathogens that take advantage of weakened hosts.
2. Opportunistic pathogens cause primary or secondary disease.

Latent Diseases

1. If host defense mechanisms fail to eliminate a microbial invader, the disease may persist as a latent disease.
2. Malaria, Brill's disease, tuberculosis, and diseases caused by herpesviruses are latent diseases.
3. Both host and environmental factors can reactivate latent diseases.

Acute, Subacute, and Chronic Diseases

1. An acute disease is a serious disease of limited duration, such as meningococcal meningitis or diphtheria.
2. A subacute disease is present before signs or symptoms are exhibited and progresses slowly; for example, subacute bacterial endocarditis.
3. A chronic disease is often mild, but persists for months or years; for example, kuru or athletes' foot.

Local and Disseminated Diseases

1. A local disease, such as most boils, remains contained at a specific site.
2. If infectious agents spread to other parts of the body, the disease is a disseminated disease; for example, coccidioidomycosis, which may be a local or disseminated disease.

Community- and Hospital-Acquired Diseases

1. Diseases in hospitalized patients are community- or hospital-acquired.
2. If a patient enters a hospital with apparent signs and symptoms of an infection, the disease is community-acquired.
3. Hospital-acquired diseases are more commonly called nosocomial diseases.

Reservoirs of Infectious Agents

1. A reservoir is a local environment or host that supports growth and multiplication of an infectious agent.
2. Humans and animals are biotic reservoirs; water, soil, and food are abiotic reservoirs.

Biotic Reservoirs

1. The reservoirs for most human pathogens are other humans.
2. Many human reservoirs show no signs or symptoms of disease.
3. Some zoonoses can be transferred to humans by contact with wild and domestic animals.
4. Certain insects and arachnids are reservoirs for protozoal, rickettsial, and other agents.

Abiotic Reservoirs

1. Soil and natural water supply nutrients that support microbial growth and multiplication.
2. Some soil pathogens produce spores if conditions are unfavorable.
3. The agents of anthrax, tetanus, botulism, and a variety of fungal diseases are soil pathogens.
4. Water is a major reservoir for agents of cholera, cryptosporidiosis, typhoid fever, amebic dysentery, and other enteric diseases.
5. The source of waterborne pathogens is improper sewage disposal or animal wastes.

Modes of Transmission

1. Infectious diseases may be transmitted by direct or indirect contact with an infected individual.
2. Persons in direct contact with infected individuals or contaminated food, water, or objects are at risk unless they have had the disease or been vaccinated against it.

Direct Contact

1. Touching, shaking hands, kissing, and sexual intercourse are forms of direct contact.
2. Molluscum contagiosum and scabies are transmitted by skin-to-skin contact.
3. Enteric diseases are often spread by contaminated hands of infected food workers or carriers.
4. Kissing provides the opportunity for an exchange of pathogens present in saliva.
5. Sexually transmitted diseases (STDs) are transmitted by intimate contact during sexual intercourse.
6. Bites of another vertebrate or arthropods transmit diseases of tropical and temperate climates.
7. Some viruses, bacteria, and protozoa are transmitted by placental transfer.

Indirect Contact

1. Intermediate materials or inanimate objects transmit diseases by indirect contact.
2. Water and food can be both reservoirs and modes of transmission.
3. Inanimate objects responsible for transmission of infectious agents are called fomites.
4. Pathogens, released into the air by coughing, sneezing, or talking, can remain suspended as aerosols and droplet nuclei.

Role of Air Currents

1. Outside and inside air currents dispense respiratory pathogens as aerosols or droplet nuclei.
2. Frequent changes of air for medical needs can be supplied by laminar flow systems.

Portals of Entry and Exit

1. Infectious agents leave the body by the same systems used as portals of entry.
2. Body fluids and waste products are vehicles of transportation for microorganisms.
3. Shedding of pathogens may continue after signs and symptoms of disease are gone.

Reporting Communicable Diseases

1. Specific communicable diseases are reported to local health agencies and forwarded to the Centers for Disease Control and Prevention (CDC) in Atlanta, Georgia.
2. Numbers of cases of illness and death due to reportable diseases are published in the *Morbidity and Mortality Weekly Report* (MMWR).
3. Annual summaries show trends, emerging patterns, and high-risk geographic areas.
4. Reports of certain communicable diseases of worldwide interest are published in the *Weekly Epidemiological Record* by the World Health Organization (WHO) in Geneva, Switzerland.

Recommendations and Regulations for Bloodborne Pathogens

1. The CDC recommends that universal precautions be followed in caring for all patients.
2. The wearing of protective garb is not complete insurance against transmission of bloodborne pathogens.
3. Extreme care must be used in handling sharp instruments or objects contaminated with blood or other body fluids.
4. OSHA regulations apply to employees who have occupational risks of exposure to bloodborne pathogens.

Study Questions for Chapter Objectives

Match a letter in column B with an item in column A. A letter may be used more than once.

Column A
___1. All communicable disease is
___2. All infectious disease is
___3. Disease produced by toxin
___4. Respiratory disease
___5. Disease is highly communicable
Column B

a. Infectious
b. Communicable
c. Contagious
d. Infectious but not always communicable

6. Define endemic disease. _____

_____

7. Define epidemic disease. _____

_____

8. Define pandemic disease. _____

_____

Quantitative Relationship

Answer *a* if *a* is larger or of greater magnitude than *b*.
Answer *b* if *b* is larger or of greater magnitude than *a*.
Answer *c* if both are about the same or if neither applies.

___9.   Number of cases of:
       a. Epidemic disease
       b. Pandemic disease

___10. Number of cases of:
       a. Endemic disease
       b. Epidemic disease

___11. The prevalence of a disease is:
       a. 12 percent
       b. 26 people ill in a group of 218 people

___12. The prevalence of a disease is:
       a. 15 percent
       b. 37 people ill in a group of 457 people

___13. The incidence of a disease is:
       a. 3.7 percent per 100,000
       b. 300 cases in 250,000 people

___14. The incidence of a disease is:
       a. 300 cases in a population of 100,000
       b. 270 cases in a population of 90,000

15. Name and describe three types of epidemiological investigations.

_____

_____

_____

_____

_____

Match a letter in column B to an item in column A.

Column A

___16. After recovery, person transmits an infectious disease agent for months and years.

___17. Person transmits an infectious disease agent without being ill.

___18. After recovery, person transmits an infectious disease agent for several days or months.

Column B

a. Carrier
b. Transient carrier
c. Chronic carrier

Calculate the incidence rate of disease Z in a small city that is growing over a three-year period, given the following information. Is the incidence rate changing in these years? How?

Disease Z	1995	1996	1997
New cases	1	8	25
Population	100,000	105,000	117,000
Incidence rate (%)	19.	20.	21.

CALCULATION SPACE for questions 19 to 21:

22. Define reservoir and give one example of a biotic reservoir and one example of an abiotic reservoir.

_____

_____

_____

_____

23. Define mode of transmission and give three examples of direct contact transmission and three examples of indirect contact transmission.

_____

_____

_____

_____

_____

_____

Match a letter from column B to a statement in column A. A letter may be used more than once.

Column A

_____24. Focus is on general population of nation
_____25. Focus is on worker population only
_____26. Establishes guidelines for safety of laboratory workers
_____27. In 1991, adopted requirements to prevent transmission of bloodborne pathogens at work
_____28. A regulatory agency of the U.S. government
_____29. A public health agency
_____30. Requires reporting of communicable diseases weekly
_____31. Receives weekly and immediate reports from physicians, and from local and state health care agencies

Column B

a. CDC
b. OSHA
c. CDC and OSHA

32. What is meant by universal precautions? _____

_____

_____

33. How do current medical practices supply portals of entry to environmental microorganisms?

_____

_____

34. Why is it important to identify disease in hospital patients as community- or hospital-acquired?

_____

_____

_____

The following chart was made from data supplied by the CDC. The graph represents results obtained in a surveillance program in seven states (A to G) in 1997. The geographic variation in penicillin-resistant strains of *Streptococcus pneumoniae* was graphed. What guidelines does this graph suggest for physicians in each state about determining suitable treatment for infections caused by *Streptococcus pneumoniae?*

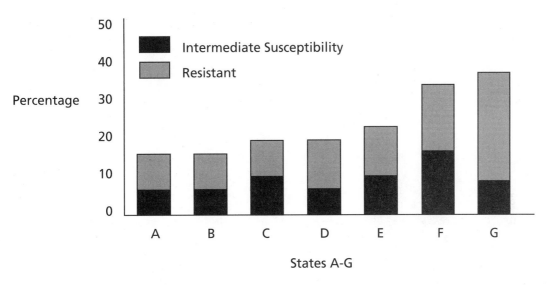

35. _____

_____

_____

_____

_____

_____

_____

_____

CHAPTER 12

The Nature of Pathogenicity

Learning Objectives

1. Differentiate between pathogenicity and virulence.
2. Describe three major factors for development of infectious disease.
3. Identify genetic factors for virulence.
4. List microbial factors responsible for virulence.
5. List host factors responsible for virulence.
6. Differentiate between exotoxins and endotoxins.
7. Define an opportunistic pathogen.

Study Outline

Determinants of Infectious Disease

1. Pathogenicity is the ability of a microorganism to cause disease.
2. The degree of pathogenicity is called virulence.
3. Invasiveness and toxigenicity permit microorganisms to injure hosts.
4. Progression of an infection to a disease depends on virulence, quantity of microbial invaders or toxins, and the resistance of the host.

Virulence

1. Virulence is not a stable characteristic.
2. Some mutations increase virulence.

Quantity of Microbial Invaders or Toxins

1. Virulence or ability of a microorganism or its toxin to do harm is measured and expressed as LD_{50}.

2. Determination of LD_{50} values is done by animal testing and may not be valid for human hosts.
3. Incubation time for a disease is determined by the quantity of an invading pathogen or toxin to which a host is exposed.

Resistance of the Host

1. Immune status is dependent on many general health factors.
2. Immune responses are often diminished by underlying disease or drug therapy.
3. Both microbial and host factors contribute to the infectious process.

Determinants of Virulence

1. Microorganisms continually develop new offense and defense strategies.
2. Host defense mechanisms are influenced by lifestyle, population density, and some practices of modern medicine.

Genetic Determinants of Virulence

1. Plasmids and bacteriophages transfer segments of DNA that carry virulence factors between cells.
2. Pathogenic bacteria carry large DNA segments called pathogenicity islands with genes for virulence factors.

Microbial Factors

1. Virulence of an organism cannot be attributed to a single factor.
2. Surface components of organelles, enzymes, and toxins contribute to virulence.

Surface Components

1. Components of capsules, pili, cell walls, and plasma membranes facilitate adherence, colonization, and antiphagocytic activity.
2. Proteins of viral envelopes or capsids bind to receptors on host cells.
3. Molecular mimicry may allow a pathogen to go unrecognized by the immune system.

Enzymes

1. Hyaluronidase, collagenase, lecithinase, and elastase destroy host tissues.
2. Kinases of some streptococci dissolve human fibrin; coagulase of virulent strains of *Staphylococcus aureus* promote clotting of plasma.

Exotoxins

1. Exotoxins are protein molecules secreted by live cells; they have specific action on particular host sites.
2. Examples of exotoxins are hemolysins, leukocidins, enterotoxins, and toxins of botulism and tetanus.

Endotoxins

1. Endotoxins are cell wall components of some gram-negative bacteria released when cells are damaged or die.
2. Most endotoxins contain a core polysaccharide, a specific polysaccharide, and lipid A.
3. Lipid A causes fever, immunosuppression, and shock.

Siderophores

1. Siderophores enable pathogens to compete with hosts for iron.
2. Limited availability of iron increases synthesis of hemolysins.

Host Factors

1. The anatomy and physiology of the human provide advantageous sites for the colonization and transit of microorganisms.
2. Small changes in the microenvironment affect the vulnerability of a host.

Skin and Mucous Secretions

1. Microbial invaders can spread across the skin faster when it is moist than when it is dry.
2. Secretions help to spread microorganisms on mucous membranes.

Adherence Factors or Host Receptors

1. Attachment of microorganisms to surfaces favors multiplication.
2. Successful colonization of a microorganism depends on both host and microbial factors.

Lymph Vessels and Nodes

1. Microorganisms entering lymphatic capillaries reach lymph nodes quickly.
2. Most microorganisms are destroyed in lymph nodes, but some viruses and rickettsias multiply in the nodes.
3. Host-microbial interactions cause tender and swollen lymph nodes.

Blood

1. Blood is an efficient transport means for microorganisms and it supplies some nutritional needs of pathogens.
2. A few bacteria and many viruses grow and multiply in lymphocytes and monocytes; malarial parasites infect red blood cells.

Cerebrospinal Fluid

1. If microorganisms enter cerebrospinal fluid (CSF), they can cross into the subarachnoid space, lining of ventricles, or spinal canal.
2. CSF is an excellent culture medium.

Nerve Tissue

1. Toxin-producing bacteria may not migrate, but toxins often travel to distant sites.
2. Bloodborne microorganisms sometimes exit capillaries in the dorsal root ganglia or travel across the blood-brain barrier into the central nervous system.

Muscle Tissue

1. All three kinds of muscle tissue support the growth of the protozoan causing Chagas' disease.

2. Some viruses can infect muscle tissue.

Peritoneum and Pleura

1. The moist surface of the peritoneum, the lining of the abdominal cavity and a covering of the abdominal organs, enables the spread of microorganisms.

2. The moist pleura lining the chest cavity and enclosing the lungs enables microorganisms to spread.

Opportunistic Pathogens

1. Immunodeficiency states provide unusual opportunities for all microorganisms to cause disease, including opportunistic pathogens.

2. Persons having severe combined immunodeficiency disease (SCID), cystic fibrosis, AIDS, or drug-induced immune impairment are vulnerable to opportunistic pathogens.

Clinical Manifestations of Disease

1. Signs are findings evident upon physical examination; symptoms are subjective complaints described by a patient.

2. A syndrome is a collection of signs and symptoms associated with a disease.

3. The four cardinal signs of inflammation are 1) heat, 2) redness, 3) swelling, and 4) pain.

 Study Questions for Chapter Objectives

List and describe three major factors for the progression of an infection into disease.

1. _____

2. _____

3. _____

Match a letter in column B with an item in column A.

Column A	Column B
___ 4. Small circular extrachromosomal DNA that transmits properties such as antibiotic resistance among bacteria	a. Pathogenicity island
	b. Bacteriophage
___ 5. Virus transfers virulence genes	c. Plasmids
___ 6. DNA segment easily moves from one part of the genome to another, introducing mutations	d. Transposons
___ 7. Large region of DNA carrying virulence genes	

Match a letter from column B identifying the organism with each virulence factor mentioned in column A. A letter may be used more than once.

Column A	Column B
___ 8. Pili	a. Human host
___ 9. Siderophores	b. Microorganism
___10. M protein	c. Both human and microorganism
___11. Receptor sites	
___12. Lymph	
___13. Flagella	
___14. Mucous secretions	
___15. Human carriers of *Staphylococcus aureus*	
___16. Lipopolysaccharide	
___17. Lectin	

18. What component of endotoxins is responsible for toxicity? _____

_____

_____

19. What triggers the secretion of siderophores by pathogens? _____

_____

_____

20. Why are the pathogenicity and virulence of so many microorganisms changeable?

_____

_____

_____

_____

21. What is meant by the blood-brain barrier? _____

_____

_____

_____

22. How do microorganisms escape the blood-brain barrier? _____

_____

_____

_____

_____

Match the toxin or enzyme in column A with the tissue or cells affected in column B.

Column A	Column B
___23. Hemolysin	a. Epidermal cells
___24. Tetanus toxin	b. White blood cells
___25. Leukocidins	c. Connective tissue
___26. Exofolins	d. Red blood cells
___27. Hyaluronidase	e. Nerve tissue

Crossword puzzle

ACROSS:

1. Subjective complaint described by a patient
5. An exotoxin that destroys red blood cells
8. Abbreviation for a measure of the lethality of a factor
10. An exotoxin that promotes the shedding of epidermal cells
11. Exotoxins consist of these types of molecules
12. Membrane lining the chest cavity and enclosing lungs
14. Degree of pathogenicity of a microorganism

DOWN:

2. An organism capable of causing disease
3. A finding that is apparent on physical examination of a patient
4. Microbial enzyme that acts on host connective tissue
6. Organic catalyst; microbial form may be virulent
7. Abbreviation for dose of a microorganism that is capable of starting an infection
9. Abbreviation for disease syndrome that results from an infection by the human immunodeficiency virus
11. Abbreviation for an opportunistic infection causing pneumonia in AIDS patients
13. Abbreviation for public health agency in Atlanta, Georgia

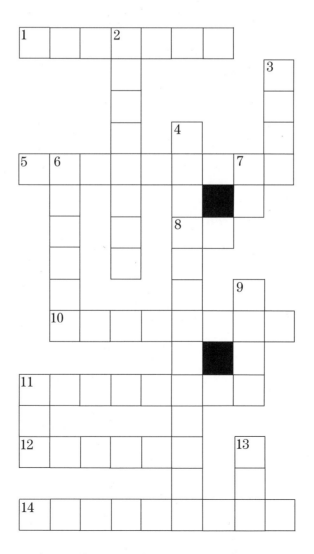

CHAPTER 13

The Immune Response

Learning Objectives

1. Compare and contrast specific and nonspecific immune responses.
2. Describe the actions of the types of leukocytes participating in immune responses.
3. Distinguish between humoral and cellular immunity.
4. Distinguish between the five classes of immunoglobulins.
5. Compare and contrast the primary and secondary immune responses.
6. Identify the roles of antigen, antibody or immunoglobulin, superantigen, cytokines, interferons, complement, B cells, T cells, macrophages, and NK cells in immunity.

Study Outline

Organs of the Lymphatic System

1. The lymphatic system is a group of organs and vessels distributed within the body.
2. The mucosal immune system is located in the mucous membranes of the intestines, respiratory system, and other organs.

Lymph Nodes, Lymph Vessels, Lymph Fluid

1. Lymph nodes contain large populations of lymphocytes.
2. Lymphocytes interact with the invading microorganisms carried to the node by the lymph fluid.

Spleen, Thymus, Peyer's Patches, and Tonsils

1. The spleen filters blood; it contains about 25 percent of the lymphocytes.
2. The thymus processes and develops mature T lymphocytes.
3. Peyer's patches are lymphatic nodules in the ileum that contain macrophages.

4. The tonsils and adenoids are mucosal lymphoid tissue protecting the oral and nasal passages against invasion.

Leukocytes Involved in the Immune System

1. The blood contains leukocytes, erythrocytes, and platelets that circulate in the plasma.
2. When blood clots, the fluid surrounding the clot is blood serum.

Origin of Blood Cells

1. Before birth, blood cells are formed primarily in the liver, spleen, thymus, lymph nodes, and red bone marrow.
2. After birth, the pluripotential stem cells in the red bone marrow produce all the blood cells.

Granulocytic Leukocytes: Neutrophils, Basophils, Eosinophils

1. Each type of granulocytic leukocyte has a specific cytoplasmic granule that secretes chemicals for defense.
2. Neutrophils, also called polymorpho-nuclear leukocytes (PMNs), are active in phagocytosis of invaders.
3. Basophils circulate in the blood; the tissue form is the mast cell; they secrete histamine or heparin.
4. Eosinophils are important in the destruction of parasitic worms and in the allergic response; they secrete antihistamines.

Agranulocytic Leukocytes: Lymphocytes, Monocyte-Macrophage System

1. The two main subpopulations of lymphocytes, the B lymphocytes (B cells) and the T lymphocytes (T cells) are major immune defense cells.
2. The monocyte-macrophage system includes monocytes that can migrate from the blood into the tissues developing into macrophages.

Platelets (Thrombocytes)

1. Platelets are fragments of megakaryocytes.
2. Blood clotting is initiated by platelets.

Innate or Nonspecific Immunity

1. Physical barriers and macrophages are two of several defense mechanisms present from birth.
2. The components of innate immunity function in any type of invasion so they are participants in nonspecific immunity.

Primary Barriers to Infection of the Body

1. The largest barriers to invasion of the body are the skin and mucous membranes.
2. Sweat glands cleanse the epithelium; apocrine cells produce fatty secretions to preserve the epithelium and inhibit growth of some bacteria.
3. The mucosal epithelium covering the eyes, respiratory, gastrointestinal, and genitourinary tracts traps microorganisms and prevents further invasion.

Secondary Barriers to Invasion into the Body

1. If the skin or mucous membranes are injured, phagocytic cells actively remove invading microorganisms.

2. Inflammation responses inhibit the penetration of deeper tissues by invading cells.

Phagocytosis

1. Macrophages patrol the tissues; they phagocytize invading microorganisms present in small numbers.
2. A large invasion activates macrophages to produce more chemicals to kill the invader.

Inflammation: Role of Macrophages, Neutrophils, and Cytokines

1. Macrophages secrete proinflammatory cytokines that attract other immune defense cells to the invasion site.
2. Cytokines attract neutrophils from the bloodstream to the site of inflammation for phagocytosis.

The Complement System

1. Complement consists of over 30 proteins that interact in a specific order in response to invading microorganisms.
2. The classical pathway is activated by antibody molecules, or by the MBLectin pathway in response to sugars in the capsules of microorganisms.
3. The membrane attack complex called MAC is a group of complement proteins that cause cell lysis.

Acute Phase Response of Liver in Inflammation

1. The proinflammatory cytokine IL-6 initiates an acute reponse by the liver.
2. The liver produces clotting factors, complement components, and other chemicals to replace those consumed during inflammation.

Role of Fever

1. Fever is a sign of inflammation; it is induced by proflammatory cytokines.
2. Fever may function to inhibit bacterial growth; it triggers the production of heat-shock proteins to enhance survival of host cells.

Interferons and Natural Killer Cells in Viral Infections

1. Interferon is a cytokine produced by a virus-infected cell, and secreted to neighboring cells to shut down metabolism that allows virus replication.
2. Natural Killer cells destroy intracellular microorganisms, tumor cells, and virus-infected cells on direct contact,

Specific Immunity

1. Only the cells and molecules specifically able to provide a defense against the specific invading microorganism are activated.
2. Memory cells are produced during each infection for rapid response to future invasions by the same etiologic agent.

Antigens

1. Antigens are large with molecular weights of 10,000 or greater; they stimulate an immune response.
2. Proteins, carbohydrates, and lipid molecules are antigenic.

Self and Nonself

1. The surface molecules on the cells, tissues, and organs of each person are self antigens; they are tolerated by the immune system.
2. Self antigens stimulate an immune response in other persons and sometimes in the person producing them in certain autoimmune disease states.
3. The antigens entering the body through contact, eating, drinking, microbial or viral invasions are nonself antigens.

Self Antigens of the Major Histocompatibility Complex

1. The proteins produced by major histocompatibility genes are cell surface antigens.
2. Two classes of major histocompatibility complex (MHC) proteins are produced by different cells: MHC class I and MHC class II.

Immunologic Tolerance

1. When lymphocytes do not become activated by foreign substances, the phenomenon is called immunologic tolerance.
2. Self tolerance is demonstrated because the immune system does not become activated by the individual person's self antigens.

Nonself Antigens

1. Antigenic molecules of microorganisms and viruses are nonself.
2. The antigenic molecules on the cells and tissues of humans and animals that serve as blood and tissue donors are nonself.

Five Classes of Antibody or Immunoglobulin Molecules

1. Antibody molecules are proteins of the gamma globulin class circulating in blood plasma and serum.
2. The five classes of immunoglobulin (Ig) molecules are: IgA, IgD, IgE, IgG, and IgM.
3. IgD, IgE, and IgG are monomeric protein molecules consisting of two heavy protein chains and two light protein chains held together by disulfide bonds in a specific Y-shaped structure.
4. IgA is a dimer, and IgM is a pentamer.
5. Each immunoglobulin molecule has two antigen-binding sites per monomeric unit; IgG has two sites, and IgM has 10 sites.
6. Immunoglobulin molecules are produced by mature activated B cells called plasma cells; they bind specifically to one type of antigenic determinant.

Phases of the Specific Immune Respone

1. The specific immune response has at least five well-recognized phases.
2. The primary immune response includes antigen recognition and presentation, activation, and effector phases, along with production of memory cells.

Antigen Recognition Phase

1. Specific receptor molecules on the surfaces of T and B cells recognize corresponding determinant units on antigens.
2. T cell receptors bind to antigen when it is bound to MHC molecules on the surface of an antigen-presenting cell such as a macrophage.
3. B cell receptors (BCRs) are a form of the immunoglobulin molecule the B cell produces; the BCR binds directly on contact with the corresponding antigen.

Antigen Presentation Phase

1. Phagocytic macrophages digest proteins of the phagocytized invader to produce peptide units.
2. The peptide units are bound to MHC molecules and deposited on the macrophage surface.
3. CD4+ T cells bind to the MHC-peptide complex on the macrophage to become activated and secrete cytokines.

Activation Phase

1. The T and B cell clones that recognize antigen are selected; they grow and divide rapidly increasing their populations.
2. Activated T cells secrete cytokines called interleukins (IL) such as IL-2 for B cell proliferation and IL-4, IL-5, and IL-6 for B cell differentiation into antibody-producing plasma cells.

Effector Phase

1. Plasma cells are effector B cells, actively secreting large amounts of immuno-globulin molecules.
2. Immunoglobulin molecules circulate in the body fluids and bind to the corresponding antigen to produce immune complexes that attract immune defense cells and molecules.
3. There are two types of CD4+ effector T cells: Th1 increases cellular immunity, and Th2 increases humoral immunity.

Primary and Secondary Immune Responses

1. The immune system response that develops the first time an antigen is encountered is called the primary response.
2. The second and subsequent encounters with the same antigen activate the memory cells in the secondary immune response.
3. IgM molecules increase in concentration early in both types of responses but declines rapidly.
4. IgG molecules lag behind IgM in the primary immune response but persist longer.
5. In the secondary response, IgG concentration increases rapidly and persists for many years of long-term protection.

Interactions of TCRs with Superantigens

1. Superantigens induce a wildly exaggerated immune response that activates tens of millions of different T cells.

2. The massive response pours large quantities of cytokines into circulation causing drastic bodily reactions such as toxic shock.

Four Categories of Acquired Immunity

1. Immunity may be acquired by natural or artificial means.
2. Natural and artificial immunity may be acquired passively or actively.

Naturally Acquired Active Immunity

1. When a person becomes ill and recovers, the protective immunoglobulins are actively produced in immune defense.
2. The IgG molecules and memory cells provide long-term protection.

Naturally Acquired Passive Immunity

1. Maternal IgG molecules cross the placenta to protect the fetus.
2. Infants are immune to the same infectious diseases to which their mothers are immune; breast-feeding transfers protective IgA molecules to the baby.

Artificially Acquired Active Immunity

1. Vaccines induce an active immune defense against the materials contained in the vaccine.
2. The IgG molecules and memory cells provide long-term protection.

Artificially Acquired Passive Immunity

1. Injections of immune globulins provide short-term protection for persons whose immune systems are damaged or stressed.
2. Rabies immune globulin is obtained from the blood of persons immunized against rabies; it is administered to persons who have been bitten by animals whose immune status to rabies is unknown.

Study Questions for Chapter Objectives

Match a letter in column B with an item in column A. A letter may be used more than once.

Column A
___ 1. IgG
___ 2. Phagocytosis
___ 3. Antigen presentation
___ 4. Plasma cell
___ 5. Inflammation
___ 6. B cell
___ 7. Intact skin
___ 8. Natural Killer cell
___ 9. CD4+ T helper cell
___10. Macrophage
___11. Red blood cells
___12. Peyer's patches
___13. Interferon
___14. Complement system
___15. Thrombocyte

Column B
a. Part of specific immune response
b. Part of nonspecific immune response
c. Not part of the immune response
d. Participates in both specific and nonspecific responses

Match a letter in column B with an item in column A.

Column A
___16. Phagocytic granulocyte
___17. Secretes antihistamine
___18. Secretes histamine, heparin
___19. Agranulocytic phagocyte
___20. Matures in thymus gland
___21. Destroys parasitic worms
___22. Produces immunoglobulins
___23. Establishes cell-mediated immunity
___24. Secretes proinflammatory cytokines
___25. Has Ig-like cell receptor for antigen
___26. Is most common WBC
___27. CD4+ cell has receptor for MHC-peptide complex

Column B
a. Basophil
b. B lymphocyte
c. Eosinophil
d. Neutrophil
e. Macrophage
f. T lymphocyte
g. Plasma cell

28. Describe humoral immunity.

_____

_____

_____

_____

29. Describe cellular immunity.

_____

_____

_____

_____

30. Of the five classes of immunoglobulin molecules, which participate in placental transfer? _____

31. Which of the immunoglobulin classes participates in opsonization? _____

_____

32. Which immunoglobulin classes are monomers? _____

33. Which immunoglobulin classes are dimers? _____

34. How many antigen-binding sites does IgG have? _____

35. How many antigen-binding sites does IgM have? _____

36. Which immunoglobulin classes are found in secretions, body fluids, blood and breast milk?

_____

37. Which immunoglobulin class is in the highest concentration in the blood? _____

_____

38. Which immunoglobulin class participates in allergy? _____

39. Which immunoglobulin class is produced early in infection? _____

40. Which immunoglobulin classes fix complement? _____

41. Which immunoglobulin class persists longest in primary and secondary immune responses? _____

42. Compare and contrast the primary and secondary immune responses.

_____

_____

_____

_____

_____

_____

_____

43. On the graph below, describe what is meant by primary challenge, secondary challenge, IgG, and IgM.

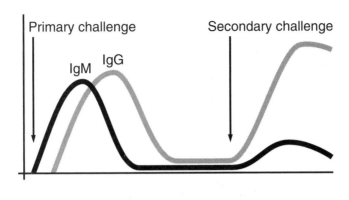

_____

_____

_____

_____

_____

44. What is responsible for the rapid secondary immune response?

_____

_____

_____

_____

45. Explain how vaccines generate immunological memory.

_____

_____

_____

_____

_____

_____

_____

_____

46. What is the part of the graph in 43 that relates to the effect of a booster dose of a vaccine? Explain your answer.

_____

_____

_____

_____

_____

_____

Match a letter in column B with an item in column A.

Column A	Column B
___47. Antigen	a. Activates tens of millions of T cells
___48. CD4+ cell	b. Group of 30 proteins, some are enzymes
___49. Superantigen	c. Produced by virus-infected cell
___50. B cell	d. Mobile, active phagocytic cell
___51. Interferon	e. Cell chemicals react with other cells
___52. Cytokines	f. Destroys tumors, virus-infected cells
___53. Macrophage	g. Stimulates immune response
___54. Complement	h. Has Ig-like receptor to an antigen
___55. NK cell	i. Recognizes antigen bound to MHC

56. On the diagram of an IgG molecule below, write in the following labels: Antigen-binding site, L chain, H chain, Disulfide bonds, Hinge region, Fc, Fab.

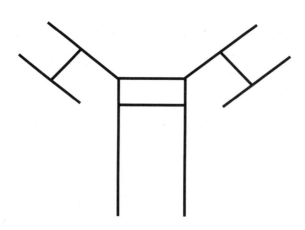

14

Alterations and Applications of the Immune Response

Learning Objectives

1. Differentiate between primary and secondary immunodeficiencies.
2. Contrast antibody- and cell-mediated hypersensitivities.
3. Explain a basic mechanism for each of the three types of antibody-mediated hypersensitivities.
4. Differentiate between immune reactions of transplant rejection and graft-versus-host reactions.
5. Describe advantages of immunological tests over cultural methods in the diagnosis of infectious diseases.
6. Explain the continuing need to provide early childhood vaccinations.

Study Outline

States of Immunodeficiency

1. Altered immune responses involving deficiencies that are present at birth are classified as primary disease.
2. If immunodeficiency disease is acquired during the lifetime of an individual, it is classified as a secondary disease.

Primary Deficiencies

1. Deficiencies in phagocytes, complement, B cells, and T cells are classified as primary.
2. The disorder may be named by the deficiency, the discoverer, or the first patient identified with the deficiency.

Phagocytic Disorders

1. Deficiencies of extrinsic activators such as cytokines or errors of metabolism of phagocytes may cause the disorder.
2. Patients with chronic granulomatous disease have an increased susceptibility to infections by bacteria and fungi with relatively low virulence.

Complement-Deficiency Diseases

1. A deficiency of complement protein C3 affects innate and acquired immunity; the patient has recurrent bacterial infections.
2. Deficiencies in complement proteins C1, C2, and C4 are characteristic of immune disorders in which patients make antibodies to self antigens.

Agammaglobulinemia and Hypogammaglobulinemia

1. These disorders are caused by a deficiency in numbers or activity of B cells.
2. Agammaglobulinemia (Bruton's disease) is linked to the X chromosome and occurs in males only.
3. Hypogammaglobulinemia may be transient, occurring in premature infants with immature CD4+ T cells, or permanent in individuals aged 15 to 35.

DiGeorge Syndrome

1. Patients have a deficiency in T cells but a normal number of B cells.

2. Transplants of fetal thymus glands can restore functioning B cells and activate CD4+ T helper cells.

Wiscott–Aldrich Syndrome

1. This disorder is a congenital combined immunodeficiency disease linked to the X chromosome; only males are affected.

2. The condition is marked by reductions in B cells, T cells, and platelets; bone marrow transplants correct these deficiencies.

Severe Combined Immunodeficiency Disease (SCID)

1. This disorder is a congenital immuno-deficiency disease linked to either the X chromosome or to an autosomal recessive gene.

2. The autosomal recessive form can be corrected by supplying the missing enzyme, adenosine deaminase.

Secondary Deficiencies

1. Following infection with the human immunodeficiency virus (HIV) destruc-tion of CD4+ T cells reduces immune responsiveness.

2. Persons who acquire immune deficien-cies during their lifetime are susceptible to opportunistic infections and malignan-cies.

B Cell Malignancies

1. An abnormal proliferation of B lympho-cytes and plasma cells and their immunoglobulins produce this type of malignancy.

2. Multiple myeloma is the most common disease associated with high numbers of plasma cells that infiltrate more than one organ system.

Autoimmune Diseases

1. Immunological self tolerance is character-istic of a healthy immune system.

2. These diseases are characterized by an attack on self antigens by the immune system.

Exaggerated Immune Responses

1. Exaggerated immune responses occur upon exposure to allergens which stimulate a hypersensitivity reaction.

2. Susceptibility to some allergens appear to be genetically-based; these are atopic allergies.

Types of Hypersensitivities

1. Hypersensitivity reactions are categorized as either immediate or delayed based on the time symptoms develop after exposure to allergen.

2. Three of the four types of hypersensitivity reactions are antibody-mediated and occur relatively soon after contact with antigen.

3. One type of hypersensitivity is cell-mediated and the symptoms are delayed, occurring hours to days after contact with antigen.

Type I Antibody-Mediated Anaphylactic Hypersensitivity

1. Anaphylactic reactions occur when allergens combine with IgE bound to the surface membrane of mast cells or circulating basophils.

2. Initial contact with the allergen results in the activation of IgE-secreting B cells, and the individual is sensitized to the allergen.

Systemic Anaphylaxis

1. The anaphylactic reaction is sudden, sometimes fatal, in response to contact with an allergen to which the person is sensitized.

2. The reaction often occurs in individuals who are allergic to penicillin or insect bites.

Localized Anaphylaxis

1. Asthma, hay fever, and urticaria (hives) are localized IgE-mediated reactions that occur after exposure to an allergen to which the person is sensitized.

2. The reactions occur in the respiratory, conjunctival, or intestinal mucosa.

Type II Antibody-Mediated Cytotoxic Hypersensitivity

1. When self antigens on blood cells or somatic cells react with IgG or IgM and complement, cell destruction or alteration occurs.

2. The antibodies promote phagocytosis.

Transfusion Reactions

1. Exposure to noncompatible antigens of the ABO blood groups in a blood trans-fusion can activate complement and circulating immunoglobulins to cause lysis of the donor red blood cells.

2. Symptoms of a transfusion reaction are pain, nausea, vomiting, low blood pressure, fever, and kidney damage.

ABO and Rh Incompatibilities of Pregnancy

1. An ABO incompatibility of maternal and fetal red blood cell antigens can promote an immune response in the mother.
2. Rh incompatibilities of pregnancy occur most frequently when the mother is Rh negative and the fetus is Rh positive for the D antigen.
3. Fetal red blood cells enter the maternal circulation just before and after delivery and activate the maternal immune system.
4. In subsequent pregnancies in which the fetus has the same noncompatible antigens, the maternal IgG crosses the placenta and causes hemolysis of fetal red blood cells.

Autoimmune Hemolytic Anemia

1. An individual develops antibodies to self antigens after exposure to drugs, infectious agents, or cancer.
2. It is believed that antigens on red blood cells are altered making them nonrecognizable as self.

Thrombocytopenia

1. Some persons produce antibodies to certain drugs or infectious agents that react with antigens on thrombocytes (platelets).
2. Complement lyses the thrombocytes and petechiae develop.

Myasthenia Gravis

1. This autoimmune disease is characterized by the presence of antibodies to acetylcholine receptors of neuromuscular junctures.
2. The disease is characterized by progressive muscle weakness, and difficulty chewing, swallowing and breathing.

Graves' Hyperthyroidism

1. This autoimmune disease is caused by antibodies that bind to antigens on the surface of thyroid cells.
2. Thyroid activity is continually stimulated; over years, the thyroid gland is enlarged producing a goiter.

Type III Antibody-Mediated Immune Complex Hypersensitivity

1. Differences between some kinds of Type II and Type III hypersensitivity reactions may be subtle.
2. Activation of complement precedes the release of chemical mediators by neutrophils.
3. Immune complexes of Type III reactions are formed in blood vessels, deposited in the vessel walls and tissues of the body causing tissue necrosis.

Arthus Reaction

1. Repeated injections of a soluble antigen in animals produces a localized reaction of inflammation and necrosis.
2. Inhaled antigens cause similar reactions in animal and human alveoli in hypersensitivity pneumonitis.

Serum Sickness

1. Proteins from animal serum were once used in the treatment of some diseases; they activated a hypersensitive response.
2. The formation of immune complexes causes painful joints, skin rash, and swollen lymph nodes for 8 to 10 days.

Rheumatic Fever

1. This disease is an active inflammatory process following a pharyngitis that is caused by some group A beta hemolytic streptococci.
2. The antibodies can cause arthritis, carditis, skin rash, Sydenham's chorea, and possibly, permanent heart valve damage.

Acute Poststreptococcal Glomerulonephritis

1. The reaction occurs within five days after a pharyngitis or a skin infection by certain group A beta hemolytic streptococci.
2. The immunologic injury causes glomerular permeability and degenerative changes in glomeruli.

Systemic Lupus Erythematosus

1. Antinuclear antibodies form complexes with antigenic components of damaged cells in the presence of complement.
2. The immune complexes deposit in small blood vessels of the heart, kidneys, lymph nodes, and synovial membranes.

Rheumatoid Arthritis

1. This disease is a chronic inflammatory disease of the joints.
2. The patient has IgM or IgG autoantibodies that react with the Fc portion of their own antibody molecules.

Polyarteritis Nodosa

1. This is an inflammatory disease of small or middle-sized arteries in which immune complexes have deposited.

2. The initial allergen may be a drug or part of an infectious agent.

Type IV Cell-Mediated Delayed Hypersensitivity

1. This response follows stimulation of Th1 and CD8+ cells by processed antigen; it occurs in the absence of antibodies.

2. The ability of some microorganisms or their products to promote erythema and induration is the basis of diagnostic skin tests such as the Mantoux test for tuberculosis.

Contact Dermatitis

1. Mild rash or erythema to weeping lesions may develop as a result of contact with some chemicals.

2. One of the most common contact allergens is urushiol found in poison ivy and poison oak.

Granulomatous Hypersensitivity

1. This is a chronic infection in which the etiologic agent lives within macrophages.

2. Continued antigenic stimulation leads to scar tissue.

Type 1 Insulin-Dependent Diabetes Mellitus

1. This condition is called juvenile diabetes.

2. Insulin-secreting cells of the pancreas are destroyed.

Multiple Sclerosis

1. Multiple sclerosis appears to be a chronic autoimmune disease of the central nervous system.

2. Characteristic of the damage is the demyelination of axons of white matter in the brain, optic nerves, or spinal cord.

Rejection of Transplants

1. Success of organ transplants is based on genetic similarities of the major histocompatibility complex between donor organs and recipient tissues.

2. The magnitude of immune rejection depends on the degree of disparity between antigens of donor and recipient.

Graft-Versus-Host Reactions

1. If immunocompetent cells of a graft react against host cells and tissues, the response is a graft-versus-host (GVH) reaction.

2. Natural killer cells from the graft secrete perforins that lyse host cells.

Applications of the Immune Response

1. Diagnosis and prevention of infectious diseases have been advanced by serological or immunological tests.

2. Rapid, sensitive, easy-to-perform tests help to identify etiologic agents that either do not grow or grow with difficulty in the laboratory.

Monoclonal Antibodies

1. Antibody-specific B cells are fused with mouse myeloma cells forming a hybridoma capable of producing large quantities of a single type of antibody.

2. Many types of immunoassays are based on using monoclonal antibodies.

Unlabeled Immunoassays

1. These tests measure antibodies in a patient's serum.

2. The tests use antigens and antibodies that are not carrying fluorescent dye labels or radioactive element labels so they are called unlabeled.

Agglutination

1. Particulate antigens react with antibody molecules producing large visible complexes that indicate a positive reaction.

2. If the antigens are on blood cells, the test is a hemagglutination.

Precipitation

1. Soluble antigens react with antibody molecules producing visible complexes that indicate a positive reaction.

2. Forensic medicine identifications of blood group antigens in blood stains depend on precipitation tests.

Complement Fixation

1. Complement binds or fixes to antigen-antibody complexes.

2. The test indicates the presence of an antigen-antibody-complement complex in a specimen when hemolysis does not occur in a sheep red blood cell-hemolysin indicator system.

Neutralization

1. The inactivation of virus or toxin agents by formation of antigen-antibody complexes in neutralization tests helps to identify the agent.

2. Toxin is neutralized by an antitoxin; neutralized virus is unable to infect host tissue.

Labeled Immunoassays

1. A fluorescent dye, a radioactive isotope, or an enzyme is attached to a molecule of antigen or antibody to produce labeled antigen or labeled antibody for use as indicator molecules in diagnostic tests.

2. Direct tests detect antigens; indirect tests detect antibodies.

Immunofluorescent Assays

1. Fluorescent dyes such as fluorescein isothiocyanate or tetramethyl rhodamine are used to label antigens or antibodies.

2. In direct testing, labeled antibody reacts directly with antigen on a smear from a clinical or tissue specimen.

3. In indirect testing, labeled anti-antibody reacts with an antigen-antibody complex to detect presence of antigen.

Radioimmunoassays

1. Radioactive isotopes are bound to antigen to produce a labeled antigen that competes with unlabeled antigen for antibodies.

2. The radioimmunoassay (RIA) method measures extremely small amounts of antigens, antibodies, or antigen-antibody complexes.

Enzyme Immunoassays

1. In direct enzyme-linked immunosorbent assay (ELISA) methods, antibodies are adsorbed to a surface, test antigen is added, followed by antibody specific for a known antigen, and an enzyme detecting system. If a color develops, the test antigen is identified.

2. In indirect ELISA, antigen is adsorbed to a surface, test serum is added, enzyme-linked anti-antibodies are added followed by the substrate of the enzyme. If a color develops, the test serum contains the antibody corresponding to the bound antigen.

Fluorescence-Activated Cell Sorting

1. Immunofluorescence and laser beam technology is used in a cell sorting device to separate and count cells in a mixture.

2. The technique is used to separate CD4+ and CD8+ cells to monitor and assess the prognosis of AIDS patients.

Western Blot Assays

1. Western blot assays are used to identify proteins.

2. The assays are used as confirmatory tests in HIV testing.

Vaccine-Preventable Diseases

1. Administration of killed or attenuated microorganisms and viruses, their parts, or inactivated toxins in appropriate dosage and schedule prevent the diseases caused by these organisms.

2. A large number of vaccines for infectious diseases affecting children and adults are available.

Study Questions for Chapter Objectives

1. Define primary immunodeficiency. _____

_____

2. List some examples of primary immunodeficiency. _____

_____

_____

3. Define secondary immunodeficiency. _____

_____

4. List some examples of secondary immunodeficiency. _____

_____

_____

5. Which of the four types of hypersensitivity are dependent on the interaction of antigens with immunoglobulins causing a hypersensitive response? _____

_____

6. From your answer in question 5, are the types called immediate hypersensitivity or delayed hypersensitivity reactions? _____

_____

7. Which of the four types of hypersensitivity are dependent on the interaction of antigens with immune defense cells causing a hypersensitivity response? _____

_____

8. From your answer in question 7, is the type called immediate hypersensitivity or delayed hypersensitivity reactions? _____

_____

9. Write the full names of the types of antibody-mediated hypersensitivity reactions and write an example of one condition for each type. _____

_____

_____

_____

_____

10. Write the full name of the type of cellular-mediated hypersensitivity reactions and write an example of one condition for the type. _____

_____

_____

Match a letter from column B to an item in column A. A letter may be used more than once.

Column A	Column B
___11. Donated organ is destroyed by recipient's immune system.	a. Transplant rejection
___12. Immune cells in tissue graft attack recipient's tissue.	b. Graft-versus-host
___13. Natural killer cells secrete perforins to lyse recipient cells.	c. Both a and b choices are correct
___14. Genetic dissimilarities are responsible.	
___15. Cell-mediated immunity is responsible.	

Match a letter from column B to an item in column A.

Column A	Column B
___16. A graft of skin from one place to another on same individual.	a. Privileged site
___17. A transplant does not generate an immune response.	b. Xenograft
___18. Tissue graft is of a different species.	c. Isograft
___19. Tissue graft is of a different individual of same species.	d. Autograft
___20. Tissue graft is from an identical twin.	e. Allograft

Match a letter from column B to an item in column A. A letter may be used more than once.

Column A	Column B
___21. IgE is involved	a. Type I hypersensitivity
___22. IgG, IgM are involved	b. Type II hypersensitivity
___23. No immunoglobulin involved	c. Type III hypersensitivity
___24. Nonself allergen	d. Type IV hypersensitivity
___25. Self allergen	e. Types II, III
___26. Complement is involved	f. Types I, III, IV
___27. Complement is not involved	g. Types I, IV
___28. Response occurs in 2-30 minutes	
___29. Response is within 24-48 hours	
___30. Anaphylaxis is one example	
___31. Transfusion reaction is one example	
___32. Mantoux skin test	
___33. Hives	
___34. Systemic lupus erythematosus	
___35. Hemolytic disease of the newborn	
___36. Prior exposure to an antigen that now stimulates Th1 cells and CD8+ cells causes erythema and induration.	
___37. Red blood cell antigens react with IgG or IgM and complement causing cell lysis.	
___38. Immune complexes deposit in blood vessel walls causing tissue necrosis.	
___39. Allergens combine with IgE on surface of mast cells.	

Match a letter in column B with an item in column A.

Column A

___40. Hybridomas produce antibodies.
___41. Blood typing uses this method.
___42. Sheep red blood cells and hemolysin are an indicator system in this method.
___43. Toxin binds with antitoxin.
___44. Forensic medicine identifies blood type of a blood stain.
___45. Radioactive isotopes identify antigen.
___46. Color reaction between enzyme and substrate is a positive result for either antigen or antibody.
___47. Fluorescent dyes detect antigen or antibody.
___48. Protein mixtures are separated and then identified by this method.

Column B

a. Western blot
b. Precipitation
c. Agglutination
d. Complement fixation
e. Immunofluorescence
f. RIA
g. Neutralization
h. ELISA
i. Monoclonal antibody

49. Explain the value of early childhood vaccinations for maintaining the public health, the health of school children and children in day care centers. Also, review the concept of herd immunity in Chapter 13 to compose your answer.

INFECTIOUS DISEASES OF HUMANS

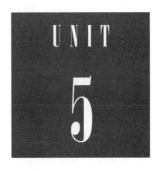

UNIT 5

CHAPTER 15

Diseases of the Skin, Hair, and Nails

Learning Objectives

1. Describe how microorganisms gain entrance through the skin.
2. Describe the lesions of the skin that are produced by infectious agents.
3. List the major bacterial, fungal, and viral diseases of the skin.
4. Contrast the treatment of bacterial, fungal, and viral infections of the skin.
5. Explain the recurrence of herpesvirus infections.
6. List the defects of congenital rubella syndrome.
7. Explain the persistence of pseudomonads in the hospital environment.

Study Outline

Introduction

1. The skin is the largest organ of the body and is composed of a layer of closely-packed epithelial cells, the epidermis, and a dense layer of connective tissue called the dermis.
2. Most of the microorganisms found on the skin are gram-positive bacteria; most gram-negative bacteria are inhibited by products of sebum degradation.

Bacterial Infections

1. Bacteria that enter the skin through an abrasion, a puncture wound, or a cut may cause a skin infection.
2. If the organisms get into the bloodstream, the infection can be life-threatening.

Acne

1. Acne is caused by the action of *Propionibacterium acnes* when it breaks down sebum and causes local inflammation and pimples.
2. Frequent cleansing of the skin and topical application of benzoyl peroxide and tetracyclines may modify acne.

Staphylococcal Infections

1. Infections caused by *Staphylococcus aureus* occur when the bacteria penetrate a hair follicle or a sebaceous gland.

2. Staphylococci cause the development of furuncles and carbuncles, examples of abscesses, and decubiti, which are open lesions from long periods of immobility.

3. Staphylococci may cause impetigo, scalded-skin syndrome, and toxic shock syndrome.

4. Toxins and enzymes produced by *S. aureus* contribute to its pathogenicity.

5. Colonization of invasive strains of *S. epidermidis* on prosthetic devices causes severe infections.

6. *S. saprophyticus* is the second most frequently isolated organism in urinary tract infections.

Streptococcal Infections

1. Most streptococcal skin infections are secondary to an infection caused by another organism.

2. Group A beta-hemolytic streptococci can cause impetigo, erysipelas, cellulitis, scarlet fever, and necrotizing fasciitis.

3. Penicillin is the drug of choice for infections caused by group A streptococci.

Anthrax

1. Anthrax is primarily a disease of cattle, goats, and sheep and is caused by *Bacillus anthracis*.

2. Cutaneous anthrax occurs in humans when they are exposed to spores of the organism, which are present in animal products including wool.

3. The virulence of *B. anthracis* is associated with capsule and toxin production.

4. Penicillin is the drug of choice for local lesions of anthrax.

Leprosy (Hansen's Disease)

1. Leprosy is an ancient disease that is still a major problem in some parts of the world.

2. The two major forms of the disease are the lepromatous form that causes nodules on the skin, and the tuberculoid form that impairs sensory responses.

3. The disease is caused by *Mycobacterium leprae,* an acid-fast bacillus, that has not been grown on artificial culture media.

4. The treatment of leprosy includes rehabilitation, education, and use of the drug diaminodiphenolsulfone in combination with other drugs.

Gas Gangrene

1. Gas gangrene is caused by a number of *Clostridium* species, but *C. perfringens* is most frequently associated with the disease.

2. A potent exotoxin called lecithinase is responsible for necrosis of infected tissue.

3. This life-threatening disease is caused by an accumulation of gas, which interferes with the blood supply to affected areas.

4. Treatment includes debridement, methicillin, streptomycin, and hyperbaric oxygen therapy.

Pseudomonas Infections

1. Pseudomonads are frequent causes of infections in postsurgical patients and people with extensive burns.

2. The virulence of *Pseudomonas aeruginosa* is caused by elastase, an enzyme that inactivates complement, and an exotoxin that interferes with the action of white blood cells.

3. Water, liquid soap, and weak disinfectants are common reservoirs for the organism in hospitals.

4. Strains of *P. aeruginosa* are usually susceptible to carbenicillin and gentamicin.

Fungal Infections

1. Fungi that cause diseases of the skin, hair, and nails are called dermatophytes.

2. Diseases that are caused by fungi are called mycoses.

Tineas

1. The superficial cutaneous infections called tinea are caused by molds belonging to the genera *Trichophyton, Epidermophyton,* and *Microsporum.*

2. Diagnosis of tinea is made from direct smears of scrapings, colony characteristics of the fungi, and macroscopic observations.

3. The only effective oral drug for treating tinea is griseofulvin; topical ointments such as miconazole and clotrimazole may be of some value.

Cutaneous Candidiasis

1. Cutaneous candidiasis is caused by *Candida* species from either exogenous or endogenous sources.

2. It occurs more often in patients who are compromised by underlying disease, an immune deficiency, or long-term antimicrobial therapy.

3. Candidiasis of the oral cavity in the newborn is called thrush.

4. Candidiasis is treated with nystatin and topical amphotericin B.

Subcutaneous Mycoses

1. The subcutaneous mycoses include sporotrichosis, the chromomycoses, and certain mycetomas.
2. If the causative fungi spread to deeper tissues, severe damage can be the result.

Sporotrichosis

1. Sporotrichosis is a chronic disease that may develop in farmers and gardeners after a puncture wound.
2. Infection follows inoculation of the spores of the dimorphic fungus, *Sporothrix schenkii.*
3. Localized sporotrichosis responds to the oral administration of saturated potassium iodide.

Chromomycoses

1. The chromomycoses are localized chronic infections of the skin and subcutaneous tissue.
2. The chromomycoses are caused by di-morphic, dark-colored fungi in the genera *Exophiala, Fonsecaea,* and *Phialophora.*
3. The chromomycoses are treated with heat in early lesions, and for later lesions, with amphotericin B.

Mycetomas

1. The mycetomas begin as subcutaneous nodules after an injury but often extend into deeper tissue.
2. At least 20 fungi and some filamentous bacteria can cause mycetomas.
3. The drug of choice for the mycetomas is dependent on the type of organism that is causing the infection.

Viral Infections

1. Some viruses are introduced into the skin primarily by abrasions, puncture wounds, and insect bites.
2. The viruses of measles, rubella, and chickenpox enter the respiratory system but spread by the bloodstream to the skin and produce lesions.

Measles

1. Measles is a highly communicable disease caused by a paramyxovirus; it is a res-piratory disease with an accompanying generalized skin rash.
2. The use of the measles vaccine has greatly reduced the incidence of measles in the United States, but outbreaks have occurred.
3. A two-dose vaccination schedule with the attenuated virus is recommended for children at age 9 months, and upon entrance to school.

Rubella

1. Rubella is a mild respiratory disease caused by a togavirus; a skin rash may develop.
2. If rubella infects a pregnant woman, severe defects in fetal development can occur and produce congenital rubella syndrome.
3. Most infants receive the rubella vaccine when they are vaccinated for measles and mumps.
4. All women of childbearing age should be vaccinated if they have not had rubella.

Herpes Simplex Infections

1. Skin infections may be caused by herpes simplex viruses (HSV) 1 or 2.
2. Lesions on the lips, which are usually called fever blisters, are commonly caused by HSV-1; lesions on the genitalia are usually caused by HSV-2.
3. Both viruses remain latent in ganglia of sensory nerve fibers and can cause recurrent infections.
4. Acyclovir is the drug of choice for the treatment of infections that are caused by either of the viruses.

Varicella-Zoster Infections

1. Chickenpox (varicella) and shingles (zoster) are caused by the varicella-zoster virus, a latent virus.
2. Chickenpox is the primary disease, and shingles is the recurrent form of the disease.
3. A rash typically occurs on the trunk and face in chickenpox, but along a single sensory nerve in shingles.
4. Acyclovir may be of value in the treatment of both diseases; a vaccine may reduce the number of cases of the disease.

Roseola Infantum

1. Roseola is caused by herpesvirus 6, which produces a self-limiting disease with symptoms of a high fever, body rash, and convulsions in infants.
2. No immunization or antiviral drug is available.

Papovavirus Infections

1. The papillomaviruses of the papovavirus group cause benign tumors known as warts on the hands, wrists, or fingers.
2. Warts may disappear with time, but if they persist, they may be removed by excision or chemicals.

Erythema Infectiosum

1. Erythema infectiosum, or fifth disease, is a mild childhood disease that is caused by parvovirus B19.

2. A rash typically occurs on the face, trunk, and extremities; no treatment or vaccine is currently available.

3. Complications include joint disease, transient inhibition of blood cell production, and fetal death.

Study Questions for Chapter Objectives

Match the type of lesion in column A with the disease in column B.

Column A	Column B
___ 1. Carbuncle	a. Anthrax
___ 2. Vesicle	b. Staphylococcal infection
___ 3. Pustule	c. Sporotrichosis
___ 4. Nodule	d. Herpes simplex infection
___ 5. Tumor	e. Papovavirus infection

Match the disease in column A with the causal agent in column B.

Column A	Column B
___ 6. Scarlet fever	a. Papovavirus
___ 7. Gas gangrene	b. Togavirus
___ 8. Toxic shock syndrome	c. *Propionibacterium acnes*
___ 9. Shingles	d. *Trichophyton* species
___10. Rubella	e. *Staphylococcus aureus*
___11. Tinea pedis	f. Group A *Streptococcus*
___12. Measles	g. Paramyxovirus
___13. Sporotrichosis	h. *Sporothrix schenckii*
___14. Warts	i. Varicella-zoster virus
___15. Acne	j. *Clostridium perfringens*

16. Describe how microorganisms and viruses gain entrance through the skin.

_____

_____

17. Name and describe five infections or syndromes caused by *Staphylococcus aureus.*

_____

_____

_____

_____

_____

_____

18. What is the role of superabsorbent tampons in toxic shock syndrome?

_____

_____

19. List the major fungal diseases of the skin, and identify the primary means of transmission of the fungus.

_____

_____

_____

_____

_____

_____

20. How can recurrences of herpesvirus infections be explained?

_____

_____

21. List the major viral diseases of the skin. _____

_____

_____

_____

_____

22. Explain the persistence of pseudomonads in the hospital environment. _____

_____

_____

23. How can decubiti be prevented in debilitated patients? _____

_____

24. What danger does rubella pose in pregnancy? _____

_____

25. List the defects of congenital rubella syndrome. _____

_____

_____

Case Study

Answer the five questions based on this description of an outbreak of disease.

Members of a garden club and state forestry workers in Pennsylvania gathered together in the spring of 1988 to participate in the annual tree distribution program. The volunteers separated conifer tree seedlings, repacked them in sphagnum moss grown in Wisconsin, and distributed the trees. Needles of the pine trees punctured the skin of some volunteers. Soon after this event, 84 people developed skin ulcers on their arms. Investigation of this outbreak of skin disease resulted in the identification of a pathogen in the skin lesions of some people, and in the bales of moss obtained from one nursery.

___26. What is the likely pathogen?

    a. *Candida albicans*
    b. *Mycobacterium leprae*
    c. *Sporothrix schenckii*
    d. *Propionibacterium acnes*
    e. Papovavirus

___27. What is the reservoir of the pathogen?

    a. Tree seedlings
    b. Sphagnum moss
    c. Sphagnum moss from one nursery
    d. Human skin
    e. Sheep wool

___28. What preventive measures could be taken in the future?

    a. Wear long-sleeved shirts
    b. Wear sturdy gardening gloves
    c. Wear protective clothing
    d. None of *a* through *c* choices
    e. All of *a* through *c* choices

___29. The disease is called?

    a. Sporotrichosis
    b. Leprosy
    c. Acne
    d. Anthrax
    e. Candidiasis

___30. What type of organism is the pathogen?

    a. Bacterium
    b. Virus
    c. Fungus
    d. Protozoan
    e. None of *a* through *d* choices

Quantitative Relationships

Answer *a* if *a* is larger or of greater magnitude than *b*.

Answer *b* if *b* is larger or of greater magnitude than *a*.

Answer *c* if *a* and *b* are about the same or if neither apply.

___31. The skin layer that contains normal skin flora is called:

    a. Subcutaneous tissue
    b. Epidermis

___32. Impetigo may involve:

    a. Staphylococci
    b. Streptococci

___33. Severe necrotizing fasciitis is associated with:

    a. *Staphylococcus aureus*
    b. *Streptococcus pyogenes*

___34. This is a highly communicable skin infection:

    a. Leprosy
    b. Impetigo

___35. Superficial cutaneous infections are called:

    a. Tinea capitis
    b. Tinea corporis

___36. This disrupts the red blood cell membrane:

    a. Hemolysin
    b. Elastase

___37. This has the capability of producing congenital disease:

    a. Rubella virus
    b. *Propionibacterium acnes*

CHAPTER 16 Diseases of the Respiratory System

Learning Objectives

1. Differentiate between upper and lower respiratory tract infection.
2. Explain the conditions that permit microorganisms to cause infection of the respiratory tract.
3. List the genera of major bacteria that cause diseases of the respiratory tract.
4. Describe the role of immunization in protecting individuals from specific respiratory pathogens.
5. Compare the endemic nature and the etiologic agents of three deep mycoses.
6. Identify the major groups of viruses that are associated with respiratory disease.

Study Outline

Introduction

1. Microorganisms become airborne as solid or liquid particles called aerosols.
2. Microorganisms of the nasopharynx somewhat reflect the microbial population of the skin.

Bacterial Infections

1. Bacteria indigenous to the oropharynx or nasal cavities, or to those bacteria contained in aerosols, may cause disease of the respiratory tract.
2. Ciliated columnar epithelial cells and alveolar macrophages prevent the implantation and colonization of bacteria in the alveoli of healthy individuals.

Staphylococcal Pneumonia

1. Staphylococci rarely cause disease of the respiratory tract in healthy adults.
2. Staphylococcal pneumonia does not usually occur in children over age 2 in the absence of a predisposing viral infection.

3. *Staphylococcus aureus,* a gram-positive cluster-forming coccus, is the most frequent cause of staphylococcal pneumonia.
4. An increasing number of strains of *S. aureus* are resistant to penicillin and methicillin.

Streptococcal Infections

1. "Strep throat" is caused by group A beta-hemolytic streptococci; it is one of the most common infectious diseases.
2. An erythrogenic toxin-producing strain of group A beta-hemolytic streptococci causes scarlet fever.
3. *Streptococcus pneumoniae,* a gram-positive chain-forming coccus, is the primary cause of lobar pneumonia in the elderly and in persons who live in closed populations.
4. Group A beta-hemolytic streptococci are usually susceptible to penicillin, but some pneumococci are multiple-drug resistant.

5. Prompt treatment with appropriate antibiotics is necessary to prevent possible serious complications.

6. A vaccine that consists of capsular material for 23 types of the pneumococcus is available for individuals at high risk.

Klebsiella Pneumonia

1. *Klebsiella pneumoniae* (Friedlander's bacillus) of capsular types 1 and 2 causes serious pneumonia.

2. The gram-negative bacillus is transmitted by aerosols or may be endogenous in patients who receive antibiotics or immunosuppressive agents.

3. Other *Klebsiella* species can cause opportunistic infections of the upper and lower respiratory tracts.

Haemophilus Infections

1. *Haemophilus influenzae,* a small gram-negative bacillus, can cause bronchiolitis, bronchitis, or pneumonia.

2. *H. influenzae* type b (Hib) causes a serious infection in children; meningitis is a common complication in young children.

3. Antibiotic therapy should be based on susceptibility tests because many strains demonstrate multiple-drug resistance.

4. It is recommended that all children receive a vaccine for a capsular polysaccharide of Hib at ages 2, 4, 6, and 15 months.

Whooping Cough (Pertussis)

1. *Bordetella pertussis,* a small gram-negative bacillus, causes whooping cough; other *Bordetella* species cause acute bronchiolitis.

2. Whooping cough is characterized by three phases: catarrhal, paroxysmal, and convalescent.

3. The use of antibiotics to affect the course of whooping cough is controversial.

4. Acellular pertussis vaccine is given in combination with diphtheria and tetanus toxoids at ages 2, 4, and 6 months; at age 15 months for the fourth dose; and at age 6 for the fifth dose.

Diphtheria

1. An exotoxin of *Corynebacterium diphtheriae* causes a severe pharyngitis known as diphtheria; the toxin may disseminate and affect the heart, kidneys, or nerves.

2. *C. diphtheriae* is a gram-positive bacillus. It is transmitted to susceptible individuals by aerosols from carriers or by infected persons.

3. Formation of a pseudomembrane in diphtheria may obstruct breathing and make a tracheotomy necessary.

4. A positive Schick test indicates susceptibility to the toxin of *C. diphtheriae.*

5. Diphtheria is treated with diphtheria antitoxin and penicillin or erythromycin.

6. Immunization with diphtheria toxoid in DTP has eliminated diphtheria as a major threat in the United States.

Tuberculosis

1. Most cases of tuberculosis are caused by the acid-fast bacillus *Mycobacterium tuberculosis,* but other species do cause similar lung disease, especially in AIDS patients.

2. Immigration from high-prevalence countries, incidence of HIV infections, and development of multiresistant strains of *M. tuberculosis* are the main factors responsible for an increase in cases of tuberculosis in the United States.

3. Mycobacteria are spread by aerosols from infected individuals.

4. Early tuberculosis may be asymptomatic, but later symptoms include a cough, fever, night sweats, and weight loss.

5. A delayed hypersensitivity reaction is the basis of Mantoux and Tine skin tests to detect exposure to the bacterium.

6. The BCG vaccine has contributed to the prevention of tuberculosis in many parts of the world.

7. Drugs used to either prevent recurrence of tuberculosis or to treat it include isoniazid, pyrazinamide, rifampin, and ethambutol.

Mycoplasmal Pneumonia

1. *Mycoplasma pneumoniae* is the cause of primary atypical pneumonia in humans.

2. The disease is spread by aerosols; it occurs more frequently in older children and young adults.

3. The paroxysmal cough and substernal discomfort of primary atypical pneumonia lasts for several weeks.

4. The drugs of choice for mycoplasmal pneumonia are tetracycline and erythromycin.

Legionellosis

1. Legionellosis is an atypical pneumonia caused by *Legionella pneumophila,* a gram-negative pleomorphic bacillus stained by a modified Gram stain that uses basic fuchsin in place of safranin.

2. *L. pneumophila* is widely distributed in nature and is dispersed by aerosols from contaminated ventilation systems.

3. The symptoms of the atypical pneumonia are fever, cough, difficulty breathing, and chest pain.

4. Erythromycin and rifampin are used to treat legionellosis.

Psittacosis (Ornithosis)

1. *Chlamydia psittaci* causes psittacosis in birds and humans.

2. The organism is transmitted from infected birds to other birds and humans by aerosols, discharges, or bites.

3. Human psittacosis may be a relatively mild disease, a severe pulmonary infection, or a septicemia.

4. A headache and a fever usually occur in early psittacosis, and a respiratory infection that is not easily distinguished from other lung infections.

5. Tetracycline is the drug of choice.

Chlamydial Pneumonia

1. *Chlamydia pneumoniae* causes an acute respiratory disease.

2. Symptoms include a productive cough, sore throat, and painful swallowing.

3. A pneumonitis caused by *C. trachomatis* is acquired by newborn infants during delivery from infected mothers.

4. Both chlamydia infections respond to treatment with tetracycline or erythromycin.

Q Fever

1. Q fever is an acute febrile influenza-like disease caused by *Coxiella burnetii.*

2. *C. burnetii* is transmitted by aerosols that contain excreta of infected animals; it remains active in soil for many years.

3. Q fever affects the lungs with little or no involvement of the upper respiratory tract.

4. Tetracycline is effective; a vaccine is available for laboratory workers or other high-risk groups.

Pulmonary Actinomycosis

1. Pulmonary actinomycosis is caused by aspiration of endogenous *Actinomyces israelii,* a gram-positive bacillus, from the pharynx.

2. Purulent or blood-streaked sputum, abscesses, and draining sinus tracts develop.

3. The hyphae of *A. israelii* are often organized into sulfur granules in affected tissues.

4. Penicillin or tetracycline are recommended for treatment.

Nocardiosis

1. Nocardiosis is a chronic disease that most often originates in the lungs.

2. The primary etiologic agent is *Nocardia asteroides,* a gram-positive pleomorphic bacillus, which resides in the soil; it is transmitted by aerosols of dusty air.

3. Early disease is characterized by a cough and fever, but the infection frequently spreads to the brain or kidney.

4. Prompt treatment with trimethoprim-sulfamethoxazole can prevent dissemination of pulmonary nocardiosis.

Fungal Infections

1. Most individuals are exposed to conidia of fungi in aerosols, but disease occurs only under special conditions.

2. The lungs are the most common sites for deep mycoses.

Histoplasmosis

1. Acute pulmonary infections caused by *Histoplasma capsulatum* occur most frequently in adult males; it is transmitted by inhalation of airborne conidia.

2. Histoplasmosis is endemic in the Ohio and Mississippi River valleys, but is not uncommon in immunosuppressed patients who live in other areas.

3. The symptoms and clinical course of histoplasmosis resembles tuberculosis; a skin test that uses histoplasmin, a protein extract from the fungus, is useful in diagnosis.

4. Amphotericin B or fluconazole are the drugs of choice.

Coccidioidomycosis

1. Coccidioidomycosis is endemic in the southwestern part of the United States.

2. The etiologic agent *Coccidioides immitis* infects many animals, grows as a mold in soil, and produces infective arthroconidia.

3. Fever develops; if a cough occurs, it may be nonproductive.

4. Amphotericin B, fluconazole or itraconazole are used in treatment.

Blastomycosis

1. Blastomycosis is an acute or chronic respiratory disease caused by *Blastomyces dermatitidis* and transmitted by inhalation of conidia in aerosols.

2. North American blastomycosis occurs most frequently in central and southeastern United States.

3. The pulmonary form of blastomycosis resembles tuberculosis and histoplasmosis in that a low-grade fever, weight loss, and a cough may be present.

4. Amphotericin B is effective against systemic blastomycosis, but ketoconazole is sometimes used to treat milder cases.

Pulmonary Aspergillosis

1. The most important pathogen that causes aspergillosis is *Aspergillus fumigatus,* which is found on decaying plants, in stored hay, and in cereal grains.

2. The organism is transmitted by inhalation of conidia.

3. Pulmonary aspergillosis has four major forms: primary acute pneumonia, formation of a "fungus ball" within a cavity, allergic form, or an opportunistic infection.

4. Aflatoxins produced by *Aspergillus* species cause serious liver disease in animals.

5. Surgical excision and administration of amphotericin B and 5-fluorocytosine may be necessary to resolve aspergillosis.

Pneumocystis carinii Pneumonia (PCP)

1. *Pneumocystis carinii* is a primary invader of the lungs in premature infants, and an opportunistic pathogen in AIDS patients.

2. The fungus causes interstitial plasma cell pneumonia, which is associated with infiltration of alveoli with plasma cells, exudate, and the fungi.

3. The drugs of choice are pentamidine and trimethoprim-sulfamethoxazole.

Viral Infections

1. Viruses may be transient residents in nasopharyngeal cells without establishing symptoms of disease.

2. Viruses cause most upper respiratory tract infections and at least half of all lower respiratory tract infections.

3. Infectious virions may be shed for varying periods after symptoms of disease have disappeared.

4. Most viruses are not susceptible to antibiotics and other chemotherapeutic agents.

Influenza

1. Influenza viruses are the primary causes of epidemics and pandemics of respiratory tract infections.

2. Types A and B influenza viruses cause cyclic outbreaks of disease throughout the world; type C almost never causes recognizable disease.

3. Influenza A can be divided into groups based on the type of glycoproteins associated with spikes of the envelope.

4. The spike glycoproteins are hemagglutinin antigens (HA), which promote clumping of red blood cells, and neuraminidase antigens (NA), which facilitate release of viruses from infected cells.

5. Symptoms of influenza include fever, chills, headache, and muscle aches one to three days after exposure.

6. Reye syndrome may be a complication of influenza in children who are treated with aspirin.

7. Administration of amantadine during the incubation period limits the duration of influenza caused by influenza virus A.

8. Vaccines rapidly become obsolete because of antigenic shift and drift.

The Common Cold

1. One of 100 or more rhinoviruses is the most frequent cause of the common cold.

2. Symptoms occur within two to three days after exposure to the virus in aerosols or on contaminated hands or fomites.

3. There is no specific treatment for the common cold.

Viral Pneumonia

1. Viral pneumonia can follow a viral infection of the upper respiratory tract or occur as a complication following surgery.

2. A number of viruses, including adenovirus serotypes 3 and 7 and respiratory syncytial virus, cause pneumonia in infants and the elderly.

3. Respiratory therapy encourages deep breathing, which is required to clear the lungs of fluid that contains microorganisms.

Hantavirus Pulmonary Syndrome

1. Hantavirus, also named Sin Nombre (no name), caused an outbreak in 1993 of a pulmonary syndrome in the "four corners" region in the southwestern United States.

2. Deer mice may be the primary reservoirs of the virus.

3. The primary mode of transmission is inhalation of aerosolized rodent saliva or feces.

4. No licensed drugs are available in the United States for treatment; ribavirin is used to treat the disease in other parts of the world.

 Study Questions for Chapter Objectives

Match the disease in column A with the etiological agent in column B.

Column A	Column B
____1. Strep throat	a. *Coccidioides immitis*
____2. Freidlander's pneumonia	b. *Staphylococcus aureus*
____3. Whooping cough	c. Group A streptococci
____4. Diphtheria	d. *Pneumocystis carinii*
____5. Leprosy	e. Influenza A
____6. Legionellosis	f. *Histoplasma capsulatum*
____7. Psittacosis	g. *Legionella pneumophila*
____8. Hantavirus pulmonary syndrome	h. Adenovirus type 3
____9. Viral pneumonia	i. *Klebsiella pneumoniae*
___10. Coccidioidomycosis	j. *Bordetella pertussis*
___11. Histoplasmosis	k. *Blastomyces dermatitidis*
___12. Influenza	l. *Corynebacterium diphtheriae*
___13. Staphylococcal pneumonia	m. *Mycobacterium tuberculosis*
___14. Q fever	n. *Mycoplasma pneumoniae*
___15. Common cold	o. *Chlamydia psittaci*
___16. Actinomycosis	p. *Coxiella burnetii*
___17. PCP	q. *Actinomyces israelii*
___18. Tuberculosis	r. *Mycobacterium leprae*
___19. Primary atypical pneumonia	s. Rhinovirus
___20. Blastomycosis	t. Hantavirus

21. Refer to the list of names in column B above. Write the letter *B* next to the names in this column that are bacterial pathogens.

22. Refer to the list of names in column B above. Write the letter *F* next to the names in this column that are fungal pathogens.

23. Name five organs that are usually involved in upper respiratory tract infections.

_____

_____

24. Name four organs or tissues that are involved in lower respiratory tract infections.

_____

_____

____ 25. Dimorphism is characteristic of all of the following fungi except which one?
   a. *Aspergillus fumigatus*
   b. *Coccidioides immitis*
   c. *Histoplasma capsulatum*
   d. *Blastomyces dermatitidis*

26. Identify the factors that contribute to the low incidence of diphtheria and whooping cough in the United States.

_____

_____

_____

27. Why does penicillin remain the drug of choice for strep throat, but not necessarily for staphylococcal infections of the respiratory tract? _____

_____

_____

_____

28. Why is it necessary to perform antibiotic susceptibility tests on strains of *Haemophilus influenzae?* _____

_____

_____

_____

29. How do the etiologic agents of mycoplasmal and chlamydial pneumonia differ from typical bacteria that cause pneumonia?

_____

_____

_____

30. List the three primary deep mycoses that affect the respiratory system. _____

_____

_____

_____

Match a letter from column B with the statement in column A.

Column A

___31. Common in Mississippi, Ohio
___32. Common in southwest USA
___33. Southeastern United States, Mississippi
     River valley
___34. Dimorphic fungus
___35. Produce deep mycoses
___36. No evidence of person-to-person transmission
___37. Amphotericin B is used to treat infection
___38. Inhaled arthrospores begin the infection
___39. Fungus is found in soil near old chicken houses, and in bat caves
___40. Organism produces a yeast-like growth on blood agar
___41. Causes a severe pneumonia in AIDS patients
___42. Symptoms and clinical course resembles tuberculosis
___43. Direct microscopic examination of sputum reveals spherules
___44. Direct microscopic examination of sputum reveals yeast cells

Column B

a. *Blastomyces dermatitidis*
b. *Coccidioides immitis*
c. *Histoplasma capsulatum*
d. All three species are correct
e. Both *a* and *c* are correct

Case Study

A college student took his visiting parents to the Anza Borrego desert in California for a long weekend. Three weeks later, his father developed fever, chest pain and a dry cough. Two days later, red tender nodules appeared on his shins, and he experienced pain and tenderness in the right ankle. A chest X-ray showed left pleural effusion. Skin testing with coccidioidin produced induration; testing with PPD showed a negative result.

___45. The most likely diagnosis is?

   a. Blastomycosis
   b. Coccidioidomycosis
   c. Histoplasmosis
   d. Tuberculosis
   e. Sporotrichosis

___46. How is this disease transmitted?

   a. Inhalation of arthrospores from dusty soil
   b. A puncture wound on the skin
   c. Inhalation of aerosolized *Mycobacterium tuberculosis*
   d. Inhalation of airborne conidia around bat caves
   e. Inhalation of *Nocardia* from dusty air

___47. The causative agent is?

   a. *Mycobacterium tuberculosis*
   b. *Coccidioides immitis*
   c. *Histoplasma capsulatum*
   d. Influenza virus Type A
   e. *Blastomyces dermatitidis*

___48. Direct examination of the father's sputum showed the causative agent by the?

   a. Thick-walled spherules with numerous endospores
   b. Slender bacterial rods that form large clumps
   c. Large spherical thick-walled yeast cells
   d. Mold hyphae, septate
   e. Bacterial cocci arranged in irregular clusters

___49. Laboratory cultivation of the sputum sample on Sabouraud dextrose agar at room temperature produced mold colonies, with hyphae displaying cells that are thick-walled and barrel-shaped called?

   a. Arthroconidia
   b. Tuberculate macroconidia
   c. Terminal or lateral conidia
   d. Multiple buds
   e. Fragmented hyphae

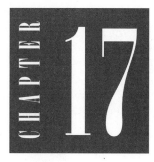

CHAPTER 17

Diseases of the Gastrointestinal Tract

Learning Objectives

1. List the major genera of microorganisms that colonize the gastrointestinal tract.
2. Discuss the causes and prevention of dental caries and periodontal disease.
3. Differentiate between a food infection and a food poisoning.
4. List the major viruses that cause infections of the gastrointestinal tract and their target organs.
5. Describe the primary features of protozoal infections of the gastrointestinal tract.
6. List methods that can be used while traveling in Third World countries to prevent gastrointestinal disease.

Study Outline

Introduction

1. The gastrointestinal tract includes organs responsible for the digestion of food, absorption of nutrients, and elimination of undigested food.
2. The accessory organs lie outside the alimentary canal and secrete or store digestive juices.
3. The normal inhabitants of the oral cavity include gram-negative cocci, gram-positive bacilli, an anaerobic *Actinomyces, Candida albicans,* and less frequently, *Entamoeba gingivalis.*
4. By being enmeshed in food particles, a few organisms escape the bactericidal action of gastric juice in the stomach.
5. The colon contains gram-positive obligate anaerobes, gram-negative facultative anaerobes, gram-positive anaerobic and aerobic cocci, and *C. albicans.*

Bacterial Diseases

1. Dental caries and periodontal disease are largely preventable by attention to diet and by the regular practice of good oral hygiene.
2. Diarrheal disease is a major cause of illness and death in developing countries.
3. Individuals with parasitic diseases are more susceptible to bacteria as secondary invaders.

Dental Caries

1. *Streptococcus mutans* is an important etiologic agent of dental caries.
2. Sucrose and other fermentable carbohydrates are cariogenic.
3. Caries are the result of demineralization of tooth enamel and destruction of dentin and cement.

Gingivitis and Periodontal Disease

1. Gingivitis and periodontal disease are caused by the accumulation of dental plaque on tooth surfaces.
2. The disease results in a progressive loss of the supporting tissues of the teeth.
3. A balanced diet and good oral hygiene can maintain the integrity of the supporting tissues, but may not prevent periodontal disease.

Salmonelloses

1. Domestic fowl are the largest single reservoir of salmonellas.
2. Three major *Salmonella* species are *Salmonella typhi*, the cause of typhoid fever, and *S. cholerae-suis* and *S. enteritidis*, which cause gastroenteritis.
3. The drug of choice for typhoid fever is chloramphenicol, but because of toxicity, it must be used judiciously.
4. The salmonellae are killed by exposure for several minutes to a temperature of 145°F (68°C).
5. Immunization with killed typhoid bacilli is recommended for high-risk groups.

Shigellosis (Bacillary Dysentery)

1. There are four major serologic types of shigellae.
2. Unlike the salmonellae, the shigellae are found only in humans.
3. *Shigella sonnei* is the most prevalent cause of bacillary dysentery in the United States.
4. Ampicillin and trimethoprim-sulfamethoxazole are often of value in treating bacillary dysentery, but antibiotic-resistant strains are increasingly common.

Travelers' Diarrhea

1. Enterotoxin-producing strains of *Escherichia coli* are one of the most frequent causes of travelers' diarrhea.
2. Two enterotoxins, a heat-labile toxin (LT) and a heat-stable toxin (ST), have been isolated from strains of *E. coli*.
3. Travelers' diarrhea is usually self-limiting, but severe cases may require fluid and electrolyte therapy.
4. Bismuth subsalicylate is effective in mild cases, but if symptoms persist, trimethoprim-sulfamethoxazole may be indicated.

Bloody Diarrhea

1. A Shiga-like toxin of *Escherichia coli* strain 0157:H7 causes severe abdominal cramps and bloody diarrhea.
2. The organism is transmitted by improperly cooked food or raw milk.
3. Kidney failure is a possible complication.
4. Antibiotic therapy is not beneficial.

Cholera

1. *Vibrio cholerae* produces a potent enterotoxin and a severe diarrheal disease known as cholera.
2. Dehydration is so severe that prompt replacement of fluid and electrolytes is required to prevent circulatory collapse and death.
3. A vaccine consisting of heat-killed vibrios is recommended for people who travel to countries where cholera is endemic.

Campylobacteriosis

1. The frequent cause of the enteric form of this disease is *Campylobacter jejuni*.
2. *C. jejuni* persists in poultry, but the organisms can also be isolated from a variety of wild and domestic animals.
3. The disease is usually self-limiting, but erythromycin is the drug of choice if symptoms persist.

Peptic Ulcers

1. The infectious nature of peptic ulcers is now recognized and attributed to *Helicobacter pylori*, a gram-negative vibrio.
2. A urea breath test is used to screen people for the presence of gastric urease, which indicates *H. pylori* infection.
3. Appropriate antibiotics eliminate the bacteria.

Gastrointestinal Yersiniosis

1. The most frequent cause of gastrointestinal yersiniosis is *Yersinia enterocolitica*.
2. The organism can be recovered from a variety of wild and domestic animals.
3. Children and young adults are particularly susceptible to the heat-stable enterotoxin of *Y. enterocolitica*.
4. The disease is either a diarrheal disease or a food poisoning.
5. Antibiotic susceptibility tests need to be performed to determine the drug of choice, since septicemia can occur.

Pseudomembranous Colitis

1. Pseudomembranous colitis occurs as a complication of antibiotic therapy.

2. The etiologic agent is an indigenous anaerobe *Clostridium difficile;* it produces potent enterotoxins A and B, which promote severe inflammatory response.

3. Vancomycin is the drug of choice.

Staphylococcal Food Poisoning

1. Staphylococcal food poisoning is caused by the ingestion of preformed heat-stable enterotoxin of *S. aureus* in foods.

2. Symptoms occur two to six hours after eating contaminated food.

3. Foods should be stored at temperatures below 40°F (4.4°C) to prevent staphylococcal food poisoning.

Botulism

1. Botulism is caused by a potent heat-labile exotoxin of *Clostridium botulinum.*

2. Most botulism outbreaks have been traced to home-canned nonacidic foods.

3. Botulinal toxin blocks the release of acetylcholine by nerve fibers; neurological symptoms occur 18 to 36 hours after ingestion of toxin.

4. Infant and wound botulism have been described in recent years.

5. Treatment of botulism consists of administration of trivalent antitoxin against types A, B, and E toxins.

Perfringens Food Poisoning

1. An exotoxin of *Clostridium perfringens* in contaminated meat and poultry is responsible for symptoms.

2. Symptoms are abdominal pain, diarrhea, and nausea within eight to 12 hours after eating contaminated food.

3. Fluid and electrolyte replacement may be necessary, but antibiotics are not indicated.

4. Thorough cooking of meat and poultry and prompt refrigeration of unused portions can reduce the risk of perfringens food poisoning.

Halophilic Vibrio Poisoning and Infection

1. Halophilic food poisoning is caused by the marine bacteria *Vibrio parahaemolyticus* or *V. vulnificus.*

2. The food poisoning is transmitted by raw or improperly-cooked seafood.

3. An explosive watery diarrhea occurs rapidly or is delayed as long as eight to 10 days after ingestion of food.

4. Control measures are aimed at keeping numbers of marine vibrios and their metabolic products below the minimal infective dose in seafood.

Viral Infections

1. In the absence of a bacterial etiologic agent, a virus is usually assumed to be the agent of gastrointestinal disease.

2. If symptoms are mild and recovery is rapid, the specific virus is almost never identified.

3. Rotaviruses and the Norwalk agent are the major causes of diarrheal disease, which is mistakenly called stomach flu.

4. Other viruses cause serious disease of accessory digestive organs.

Mumps

1. Mumps is an acute infection of the parotid glands that is caused by a paramyxovirus; it is spread from an infected person by oral or respiratory secretions.

2. The virus can spread and affect a variety of organs, including the brain and testicles, and may lead to sterility.

3. There is no specific antiviral drug for mumps; an attenuated mumps virus vaccine has reduced disease incidence.

Cytomegalovirus Infection

1. Cytomegalovirus (CMV) is a herpesvirus that causes colitis, esophagitis, gastritis, and hepatitis.

2. The virus is transmitted by placental transfer, but may be acquired throughout life by direct contact with an infected person, blood, or organ transplants.

3. CMV infection is a frequent complication in AIDS patients.

4. No antiviral drug is effective for gastrointestinal CMV disease.

Hepatitis

1. The most common forms of hepatitis are caused by hepatitis viruses A (HAV), B (HBV), and C (HCV).

2. HAV is a picornavirus transmitted by food and water; HBV is a hepadnavirus transmitted parenterally.

3. HCV resembles the flaviviruses and is transmitted parenterally or by water.

4. Hepatitis A is usually milder than the other two forms of hepatitis.

5. Jaundice may occur in all three forms of the disease.

6. A particle known as the delta agent is a defective virus that replicates only in the presence of HBV.

7. Hepatitis E virus (HEV) is the cause of waterborne epidemics in developing countries.

8. Interferons are used to treat HBV and HCV infections; immune serum globulin may reduce symptoms of hepatitis A.

9. A vaccine for HAV is available; a vaccine for HBV is recommended for high-risk groups and children.

Algal and Fungal Toxin-Associated Disease

1. Some cyanobacteria, eucaryotic algae, and fungi cause toxin-associated disease in animals and in humans.

2. Blooms of the cyanobacterium *Anabaena* have caused serious wildlife and livestock poisonings.

3. Moldy grains are responsible for food poisoning and tumors in animals; the role of mycotoxins in human disease is less established.

Protozoal Infections

1. Pathogenic protozoa have been significant causes of diarrhea and dysentery throughout history.

2. It is likely that protozoa caused diarrheal disease and decimated entire troops during wars.

Amebiasis (Amebic Dysentery)

1. *Entamoeba histolytica* is the primary cause of amebiasis.

2. Most amebiasis is transmitted by ingestion of food or water containing cysts of the ameba.

3. Trophozoites colonize the large intestine, but can disseminate to the brain, liver, and lungs.

4. The dysenteric form of amebiasis is accompanied by ulceration of the lining of the large intestine.

5. Infections of the intestinal lumen are treated with iodoquinol and diloxanide furoate; invasive amebiasis is treated by metronidazole, chloroquine, and emetine.

Giardiasis

1. Giardiasis is an infection of the duodenum or jejunum caused by the flagellate, *Giardia lamblia.*

2. Giardiasis is most often transmitted by food or water contaminated with cysts.

3. Acute giardiasis may be self-limiting, but the chronic form of the disease may last for years.

4. Metronidazole, furazolidone, or quinacrine eradicates the protozoan from the small intestine.

Balantidiasis

1. *Balantidium coli* is the only pathogenic ciliate that causes dysentery in humans.

2. The disease is transmitted by ingestion of food or water containing cysts.

3. Pigs are the most important reservoir of *B. coli.*

4. Balantidiasis can take a rapidly fulminating course in immunocompromised individuals.

5. Tetracycline is the drug of choice for balantidiasis.

Cryptosporidiosis

1. Cryptosporidiosis has surfaced in the last decade as a cause of human disease.

2. The oral-fecal route is the most probable mode of transmission of the oocysts of *Cryptosporidium parvum.*

3. Cryptosporidiosis is a frequent opportunistic infection in AIDS patients.

4. No effective treatment is available for cryptosporidiosis.

Study Questions for Chapter Objectives

1. List the major genera of microorganisms that colonize the oral cavity and oropharynx.

   _____

   _____

   _____

2. List the major genera of microorganisms that colonize the intestinal tract.

   _____

   _____

3. List the major viruses that cause infections of the gastrointestinal tract, and identify the usual target organ for each virus. _____

   _____

   _____

4. Explain how microorganisms escape the action of gastric juice in the stomach.

   _____

   _____

Match a letter from column B with an organism in column A to identify the relationship of the organism to the gastrointestinal tract.

Column A	Column B
____5. *Clostridium perfringens*	a. Indigenous
____6. *Yersinia enterocolitica*	b. Pathogenic
____7. *Escherichia coli*	c. Both *a* and *b* choices
____8. *Campylobacter jejuni*	d. Neither *a* nor *b* choices
____9. *Clostridium difficile*	
___10. *Salmonella enteritidis*	
___11. *Streptococcus mutans*	
___12. *Salmonella typhi*	
___13. *Shigella sonnei*	
___14. *E. coli* 0157:H7	
___15. *Vibrio cholerae*	

16. Explain how botulism is classified as a food poisoning rather than a food infection.

_____

_____

17. Describe what is meant by a food infection. _____

_____

_____

18. Describe what is meant by a food poisoning. _____

_____

_____

19. List some precautions for preventing gastrointestinal disease that a person can take while traveling in a Third World country.

_____

_____

_____

_____

_____

_____

Write in the scientific name of an etiologic agent for each of the following diseases.

20. Gastrointestinal yersiniosis: _____

21. Pseudomembranous colitis: _____

22. Amebiasis: _____

23. Campylobacteriosis: _____

24. CMV infection: _____

25. Bacillary dysentery: _____

26. Mumps: _____

27. Halophilic food poisoning: _____

28. Hepatitis: _____

29. Botulism: _____

30. Cholera: _____

31. Typhoid fever: _____

32. Giardiasis: _____

33. Travelers' diarrhea: _____

34. Bloody diarrhea: _____

Quantitative Relationships

Answer *a* if a is larger or of greater magnitude than *b*.

Answer *b* if b is larger or of greater magnitude than *a*.

Answer *c* if both are about the same or if neither apply.

___35. This disease involves more tissue damage:
   a. Gingivitis
   b. Periodontal disease

___36. Bacteria commonly transmitted by contaminated eggs and poultry:
   a. Salmonellas
   b. Shigellas

___37. Pathogen causes ulcerations to develop:
   a. *Helicobacter pylori*
   b. *Clostridium difficile*

___38. Toxin is more stable when boiled:
   a. Botulinal toxin
   b. Staphylococcal enterotoxin

___39. Jaundice develops within a few days:
   a. Hepatitis A infection
   b. Hepatitis B infection

___40. Can transmit halophilic vibrio infections:
   a. Raw fish on sushi
   b. Raw oysters, inadequately-cooked crab, shrimp, clams, and scallops

Fill in the appropriate answer in the table below:

Disease Agent	Target Organ	Transmission Mode
41. Hepatitis A virus		
42. Mumps virus		
43. Cytomegalovirus		

Crossword Puzzle:

ACROSS

1. Soft tissue that surrounds the teeth
5. Prefix means chain-forming, as in cocci
7. Suffix means inflammation
9. Cariogenic carbohydrate
12. Thin layer of bone below gumline
13. Tissue, bone surrounding teeth
14. Pertaining to mouth

DOWN

2. Cariogenic species of *Streptococcus*
3. A method to remove plaque
4. Decay of tooth enamel
6. Bacteria, food adhere to tooth
8. Condition of gum in gingivitis
10. Calcium, minerals form tooth layer
11. Anaerobic filamentous bacteria in plaque, ends in -*myces*

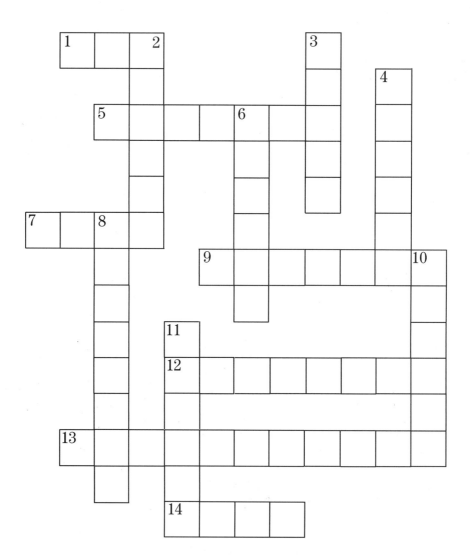

CHAPTER 18

Diseases of the Genitourinary Tract

Learning Objectives

1. Explain why urinary tract infections are more common in women than in men.
2. Name the most common isolates of urinary tract infections.
3. Name several bacteria associated with pelvic inflammatory disease.
4. Explain the significance of penicillinase-producing *Neisseria gonorrhoeae* and chromosomally-mediated resistant *N. gonorrhoeae*.
5. Name one fungus and one protozoan that cause vaginitis.
6. Explain why genital herpes infections may be of exogenous or endogenous origin.

Study Outline

Introduction

1. The anatomic proximity of the urinary and genital systems provides the opportunity for microorganisms to invade both systems.
2. The indigenous microorganisms of the distal urethra include those of the skin and those of intestinal origin.
3. The microbial flora of the vagina varies with age and during the menstrual cycle.

Bacterial Infections

1. Urinary tract infections occur in women about 30 times more frequently than in men.
2. The shorter urethra in females, moisture, and injury occurring during intercourse provide conditions for infection.
3. Sexually transmitted diseases (STDs) are the most serious infections of the genital tract.

Nongonococcal Urethritis

1. *Chlamydia trachomatis* causes about half of all nongonococcal urethritis (NGU).
2. Other bacteria that cause NGU are staphylococci, streptococci, mycoplasmas, ureaplasmas, gram-negative cocci, and gram-negative bacilli.
3. NGU requires prompt treatment to prevent ascending urinary tract infection.

Urinary Tract Infections

1. Urinary tract infections (UTI) are usually caused by gram-negative enteric bacteria such as *Escherichia coli*.
2. Some anaerobes act synergistically to cause UTI.
3. Retention of urine in the bladder and poor hygiene habits contribute to UTI.

Leptospirosis

1. Leptospirosis is a multisystem disease that frequently affects the kidneys.

2. *Leptospira interrogans,* serotype *icterohaemorrhagiae,* causes the most serious disease.

3. Dogs are the major source of human leptospirosis.

4. The drugs of choice are penicillin and tetracycline.

Pelvic Inflammatory Disease

1. Most pelvic inflammatory disease (PID) occurs in sexually-active women of child-bearing age.

2. Most cases of PID in the United States are caused by either *Chlamydia trachomatis* or *Neisseria gonorrhoeae.*

3. *Bacteroides fragilis* is the most commonly isolated anaerobe in PID; mixed infections sometimes occur.

4. Broad-spectrum antibiotics are recommended for treatment of PID.

Nonspecific Vaginitis

1. Nonspecific vaginitis is usually caused by anaerobes and the bacterium *Gardnerella vaginalis.*

2. Stippled or granular epithelial cells in vaginal fluid, called "clue cells," indicate the presence of *Gardnerella vaginalis.*

3. The infection is treated by metronidazole and other drugs.

Group B Streptococcal Infection

1. Group B streptococci (GBS) or *Streptococcus agalactiae* colonize the vagina of 15 to 20 percent of pregnant women.

2. Contamination of amniotic fluid with GBS puts infants at risk for developing sepsis, pneumonia, or meningitis.

3. GBS are usually detected late in pregnancy or during labor.

4. Ampicillin is the drug of choice for mothers and infants.

Chlamydial Infections

1. Genital chlamydial infections are the most common STDs in the United States.

2. Common complications are ectopic pregnancy and infertility.

3. Newborns can experience conjunctivitis or pneumonia if *C. trachomatis* is transmitted during a vaginal delivery.

4. Tetracycline, azithromycin, or erythromycin is used to treat chlamydial infections.

Gonorrhea

1. Gonorrhea is one of the most prevalent STDs.

2. The etiologic agent, *Neisseria gonorrhoeae,* invades epithelial tissue of the urogenital tract in adults, and the conjunctiva in adults and infants.

3. Complications include urethral stricture, sterility, ectopic pregnancy, arthritis, and peritonitis.

4. Installation of prophylactic agents in the eyes of newborns is required by most states to prevent ophthalmia neonatorum.

5. The emergence of penicillinase-producing *N. gonorrhoeae* (PPNG) and chromosomally-mediated tetracycline-resistant *N. gonorrhoeae* strains have made spectinomycin, ceftriaxone, and ciprofloxacin the drugs of choice.

Syphilis

1. Syphilis is an acute or chronic infection caused by *Treponema pallidum,* a spirochete.

2. Primary syphilis is characterized by a chancre that appears 10 to 90 days after exposure to *T. pallidum.*

3. A rash is a prominent feature of secondary syphilis.

4. In untreated cases, the period prior to or following secondary syphilis is described as a latent stage in which there are no apparent signs of infection.

5. The tertiary stage is characterized by internal lesions called gummas, neurological dysfunction, and cardiac disorders.

6. Congenital syphilis can cause death or developmental abnormalities in the fetus.

7. Penicillin is the drug of choice.

Chancroid

1. Chancroid is characterized by an ulcer known as a soft chancre, which may be confused with lesions of syphilis or herpes simplex infection.

2. The etiologic agent is *Haemophilus ducreyi.*

3. Azithromycin is used in a single-dose treatment.

Lymphogranuloma Venereum

1. Lymphogranuloma venereum (LGV) is caused by some strains of *Chlamydia trachomatis.*

2. Initial lesions are followed by enlargement of lymph nodes, known as buboes, in the groin.

3. Erythromycin, sulfamethoxazole, or tetracycline is used to treat LGV.

Granuloma Inguinale

1. Granuloma inguinale is an ulcerative genital infection caused by *Calymmatobacterium granulomatis*.

2. The disease is endemic in tropical and subtropical climates, but it is not highly communicable.

3. The drug of choice is ampicillin or tetracycline.

Fungal Infections

1. Colonization of the vagina by yeast is favored by the acidity of the vagina.

2. Fungal infections of the genitourinary tract are rare, except for those caused by *Candida albicans*.

Vulvovaginal Candidiasis

1. Vulvovaginal candidiasis is most frequently caused by *Candida albicans*.

2. The infection is common in diabetics, in women during pregnancy, and in women who take corticosteroids or broad-spectrum antibacterial drugs.

3. Most infections are endogenous in origin.

4. Miconazole or nystatin are used to treat vulvovaginal candidiasis.

Protozoal Infections

1. Most pathogenic protozoa grow well in intestines or blood.

2. An exception is *Trichomonas vaginalis,* which may be indigenous to the vagina.

3. The protozoa can cause urethritis, cystitis, or vaginitis.

Trichomoniasis

1. Trichomoniasis may occur as a single infection or may coexist with candidiasis in the vagina.

2. The etiologic agent *Trichomonas vaginalis* is a flagellated protozoan.

3. Metronidazole is the drug of choice.

Viral Infections

1. Many sexually transmittable viruses probably reside undetected in the genitourinary tract.

2. Viruses of mumps, rubeola, and cytomegalovirus disease are shed in urine.

3. The human immunodeficiency virus (HIV) is shed in semen and cervical secretions.

Genital Herpes Infection

1. Most genital herpes infections are caused by herpes simplex virus type 2 (HSV-2), but increasingly, herpes simplex virus type 1 (HSV-1) causes genital infections.

2. The disease can occur as a primary exogenous infection or as a recurrent endogenous infection.

3. The lesions of genital herpes infections are painful and often accompanied by fever, dysuria, and swelling of lymph nodes in the groin.

4. Acyclovir may alleviate some symptoms and shorten the course of primary genital herpes infections.

Genital Warts (Condyloma Acuminata)

1. Genital warts are caused by six types of papillomaviruses.

2. Warts may occur on external or internal parts of the genitourinary system.

3. Genital warts have been linked to squamous cell genital cancer, so Pap smears are recommended to detect cell changes.

4. Treatment consists of freezing, electro-surgery, laser vaporization, or podophyllin.

5. No form of treatment prevents recurrences.

Acquired Immunodeficiency Syndrome

1. Acquired immunodeficiency syndrome (AIDS) is classified as an STD, but the human immunodeficiency virus (HIV) that causes AIDS, infects CD4+ T cells of the immune system.

2. Symptoms of other STDs persist longer in individuals who are also infected with HIV.

3. Other STDs may be risk factors in the heterosexual transmission of HIV.

Study Questions for Chapter Objectives

1. Explain why urinary tract infections are more common in women than in men.

   _____

   _____

   _____

2. List the most commonly isolated microorganisms in urinary tract infections.

   _____

   _____

   _____

3. List three bacteria that cause pelvic inflammatory disease.

   _____

   _____

   _____

4. Name a fungus and a protozoan that cause vaginitis.

   _____

   _____

   _____

5. Explain what is meant by exogenous infection. _____

   _____

6. Explain what is meant by endogenous infection. _____

   _____

7. Explain how genital herpes may be exogenous and endogenous in origin.

   _____

   _____

   _____

Match each lesion in column A with an STD in column B.

Column A

___8. Bullae

___9. Nodule

___10. Chancre

___11. Gumma

___12. Bubo

___13. Corneal ulcer

Column B

a. Ophthalmia neonatorum

b. Primary syphilis

c. Lymphogranuloma venereum

d. Granuloma inguinale

e. Tertiary syphilis

f. Congenital syphilis

___14. Which antibiotic is the treatment of choice for syphilis?

a. Erythromycin
b. Tetracycline
c. Penicillin
d. Ceftriaxone
e. Doxycycline

___15. Penicillinase-producing *Neisseria gonorrhoeae* infections are treated by which antibiotics?

a. Ceftriaxone
b. Cefixime
c. Ciprofloxacin
d. Penicillin
e. One or more of *a* through *c* choices

___16. Chromosomally-mediated resistant *Neisseria gonorrhoeae* infections are not susceptible to which antibiotic?

a. Penicillin
b. Tetracycline
c. Ceftriaxone
d. Cefixime
e. Ciprofloxacin

___17. PPNG and TRNG strains of *Neisseria gonorrhoeae* are usually susceptible to which antibiotic?

a. Penicillin
b. Tetracycline
c. Ceftriaxone
d. Erythromycin
e. All of *a* through *d* choices

Quantitative Relationships

Answer *a* if a is larger or of greater magnitude than *b*.

Answer *b* if b is larger or of greater magnitude than *a*.

Answer *c* if both are about the same or if neither apply.

___18. Symptoms of gonorrhea are obvious and easy to detect in:

a. Men
b. Women

___19. Gonococcal arthritis can occur in:

a. Women
b. Men

___20. Sterility is a complication of gonorrhea in:

a. Women
b. Men

___21. The most prevalent STD in the world is:

a. Syphilis
b. Gonorrhea

___22. Transmission of gonorrhea is primarily by:

a. Sexual intercourse
b. Toilet seat

___23. Gram stains are used to detect polymorphonuclear neutrophils that contain gram-negative diplococci in:

a. Urethral exudates
b. Cervical exudates

___24. Cultures are more reliable for diagnosing gonorrhea in:

a. Men
b. Women

___25. The most frequent cause of urinary tract infections is?

   a. *Escherichia coli*
   b. Staphylococci
   c. Streptococci
   d. *Bacteroides*
   e. *Enterococcus faecium*

___26. Nongonococcal urethritis is caused by?

   a. *Neisseria gonorrhoeae*
   b. *Chlamydia trachomatis*
   c. *Mycoplasma genitalium*
   d. *Ureaplasma urealyticum*
   e. All except choice *a*

___27. The most common spirochete that causes kidney infection is?

   a. Leptospira interrogans serotype icterohaemorrhagiae
   b. *Mycobacterium leprae*
   c. *Escherichia coli*
   d. *Staphylococcus aureus*
   e. *Borrelia recurrentis*

___28. Pelvic inflammatory disease is most common in?

   a. Postmenopausal women
   b. Sexually active men
   c. Menopausal women
   d. Sexually active women of child-bearing age
   e. None of the *a* through *d* choices

___29. Organisms that cause pelvic inflammatory disease are?

   a. Anaerobic gram-negative cocci and bacilli
   b. *Bacteroides fragilis* and other anaerobes
   c. *Chlamydia trachomatis* and *Neisseria gonorrhoeae*
   d. Anaerobic gram-positive cocci and bacilli
   e. All of *a* through *d* choices

___30. Which organisms are responsible for infections of the newborn infant even when no infection is detected in the mother?

   a. Group B streptococci
   b. *Streptococcus agalactiae*
   c. *Streptococcus pneumoniae*
   d. Choices *a* and *b* are correct
   e. All *a* through *c* choices are correct

___31. The lesion of primary syphilis may be mistaken for what other STDs?

   a. Herpes simplex virus
   b. *Haemophilus ducreyi*
   c. *Neisseria gonorrhoeae*
   d. Choices *a* and *b* are correct
   e. All *a* through *c* choices are correct

___32. Vulvovaginitis of endogenous origin is usually caused by which species?

   a. *Staphylococcus aureus*
   b. *Streptococcus pneumoniae*
   c. *Candida albicans*
   d. *Cryptococcus neoformans*
   e. *Neisseria gonorrhoeae*

33. Name the lesions and describe the symptoms that characterize primary, secondary, tertiary, and latent stages of syphilis.

34. Explain the role of chlamydias and mycoplasmas in genitourinary tract infections.

_____

_____

_____

Write the name of one etiologic agent for each of the following diseases:

35. Chancroid: _____

36. Granuloma inguinale: _____

37. Lymphogranuloma venereum: _____

38. Trichomoniasis: _____

39. Syphilis: _____

40. Genital herpes infection: _____

41. Acquired immunodeficiency syndrome: _____

42. Nongonococcal urethritis: _____

43. Vulvovaginal candidiasis: _____

44. Nonspecific vaginitis: _____

45. Pelvic inflammatory disease: _____

46. Leptospirosis: _____

47. Genital warts: _____

Case Study

A 22-year old man arrived at his local public health department's STD clinic with a two-day history of purulent urethral discharge. He reported having had multiple female sex partners. Two weeks before he arrived at the STD clinic, he had one sexual encounter with an unknown woman from the United States whom he met in a nightclub frequented by U.S. military personnel in Tijuana, Mexico. He also had a steady sex partner of seven months.

___48. Gram-negative intracellular diplococci were detected in the urethral discharge indicating?

a. Syphilis
b. Chlamydia
c. Gonorrhea
d. Trichomoniasis
e. Candidiasis

___49. His steady sex partner was tested for the same infection; the results were negative, but she was given treatment because?

a. She is resistant to the disease.
b. She may not yet show symptoms of the disease.
c. She has some other genital infection.
d. She is not the source of his infection.
e. None of *a* through *d* choices

___50. The patient was treated with ofloxacin and doxycycline, but not penicillin because of which strains that cause disease?

a. PPNG
b. TRNG
c. Both *a* and *b* choices
d. Neither *a* nor *b* choices

___51. The diagnosis was confirmed by which laboratory tests?

a. Incubation at 35°C with 3 to 10 percent CO_2 on modified Thayer-Martin agar
b. Oxidase positive colonies
c. Carbohydrate fermentation results
d. All of *a* through *c* choices
e. None of *a* through *c* choices

___52. The patient was asked for the names of his sex partners because?

a. Health department follow up is necessary.
b. To notify the partners of a possible infection.
c. To provide testing and treatment.
d. All of *a* through *c* choices
e. None of *a* through *c* choices

Diseases of the Nervous System, Eye, and Ear

Learning Objectives

1. Describe how microorganisms gain entrance to neural tissue.
2. List the bacteria that commonly cause meningitis.
3. List the major microbial diseases and etiologic agents of eye and ear infections.
4. List the major fungi and protozoa that cause diseases of the nervous system.
5. Explain how central nervous system diseases that are believed to be caused by prions differ from viral infections of the central nerous system.

Study Outline

Introduction

1. The central and peripheral nervous systems are normally sterile.
2. The indigeneous microorganisms of the conjunctiva and the external auditory canal are largely a reflection of those found on the skin.
3. Microorganisms and some antibiotics in the blood have difficulty in entering the brain and meninges because of the selective permeability of their capillaries.
4. In severe septicemia, even intact blood and cerebrospinal fluid barriers do not prevent microorganisms from migrating to neural tissue.
5. Microorganisms and their toxins can reach the central nerous system by way of the eustachian tube, mastoid process, peripheral nerves, or cribriform plate, or by trauma.
6. The conjunctiva, eyelid, and bactericidal activity of lysozyme protect the eye from invading microorganisms.

Bacterial Infections

1. Most bacterial diseases of the nervous system involve the meninges by causing inflammation of the pia mater and the arachnoid.
2. The etiologic agents are frequently detected in the cerebrospinal fluid (CSF).

Meningococcal Meningitis

1. Meningococcal meningitis is caused by *Neisseria meningitidis* and is transmitted by aerosols or nasopharyngeal discharges from an infected person or carrier.
2. Symptoms include an abrupt onset of fever and nausea which may progress to vomiting, stiff neck, and small hemorrhagic spots on the skin known as petechiae.
3. The disease may culminate in adrenal hemorrhage and adrenal collapse within 24 hours.
4. Penicillin is the drug of choice.

5. Monovalent vaccines of purified capsular polysaccharides A and C and a bivalent A-C vaccine are available; vaccines are given routinely to military recruits who live and work in close quarters.

Haemophilus Meningitis

1. The most common cause of meningitis in young children is *Haemophilus influenzae* type B (HIB).
2. The organism is transmitted by contact with nasopharyngeal discharges from an infected person or carrier.
3. The symptoms, which include fever, vomiting, stiff neck, and lethargy, may follow otitis media or sinusitis.
4. The drugs of choice are ampicillin and chloramphenicol.
5. Hib capsular polysaccharide vaccine is recommended for children ages 2 to 5 months.

Streptococcal Meningitis

1. *Streptococcus pneumoniae* is the third most common cause of bacterial meningitis, and its symptoms are indistinguishable from other types of meningitis.
2. Streptococcal meningitis is frequently a complication of other pneumococcal infections.
3. Penicillin is the drug of choice.

Other Bacterial Meningitides

1. Most meningitis that is caused by other bacteria is an extension of a primary infection or the result of a brain or spinal cord injury.
2. Group B streptococci and *Listeria monocytogenes* cause meningitis in newborns because of congenital transmission of the bacteria.
3. Penicillin, ampicillin, and tetracycline may be used to treat bacterial meningitis of an unknown etiology.

Brain Abscess

1. A brain abscess is a pyogenic local infection of the brain.
2. The infection can be an extension of a primary infection or the result of trauma.
3. Most brain abscesses that stem from a primary infection are caused by anaerobes.
4. Surgical intervention and the administration of penicillin, chloramphenicol, metronidazole, or other drugs are often used.

Tetanus

1. Tetanus is a severe disease that is a complication of a wound infected with *Clostridium tetani.*
2. The exotoxin of *C. tetani* spreads along axons to the central nerous system and causes muscle rigidity, paralysis, and death in unprotected individuals.
3. Treatment consists of tetanus immune globulin (TIG) and supportive care.
4. Maximum protection against tetanus begins in infancy when tetanus toxoid is injected three times as a part of DTaP (diptheria toxoid, tetanus toxoid, acellular pertussis vaccine) shots. The fourth and fifth DTaP shots are given at 15 months and age five years to complete childhood immunization. To maintain protection, tetanus toxoid shots are necessary every ten years.

Conjunctivitis

1. Conjunctivitis can be caused by a variety of organisms.
2. Transmission is by contaminated fingers, linens, or other articles.
3. Newborn infants can acquire the infection from their mothers during delivery.
4. The drugs of choice are broad-spectrum antibiotics, penicillinase-resistant penicillins, and aminoglycosides.

Trachoma

1. Trachoma is a chronic form of conjunctivitis caused by *Chlamydia trachomatis.*
2. *C. trachomatis* is transmitted during contact with ocular or nasal discharges from an infected individual, or by contaminated materials.
3. If untreated, trachoma causes a progressive loss of vision followed by blindness.
4. Topical erythromycin or penicillin is used to prevent and treat trachoma.

Otitis Media

1. Otitis media is an acute or chronic inflammation of the middle ear.
2. Acute otitis media occurs frequently in children.
3. The disease is caused by the upward migration of nasopharyngeal bacteria through the eustachian tube.
4. Complications include mastoiditis, meningitis, and brain abscess.
5. The drugs of choice are penicillinase-resistant penicillins and erythromycin.

Fungal Infections

1. Infections of the nervous system, eye, or ear that are caused by fungi typically occur in the immunocompromised host.

2. The presence of underlying degenerative disease predisposes some individuals to fungal infections.

3. The infections are almost always fatal.

Cryptococcosis

1. The primary site of cryptococcosis is usually the lung.

2. The etiologic agent, *Cryptococcus neoformans,* is worldwide in distribution; exposure to pigeon droppings is the most important factor in transmission of *C. neoformans.*

3. Extension of the infection to the meninges causes meningoencephalitis.

4. Chronic cryptococcosis may be present for 10 to 20 years, but if untreated, it is more often a rapid, fulminating disease with a mortality rate of 100 percent.

5. Amphotericin B, fluconazole, and flucytosine are the drugs of choice.

Cerebrorhinoorbital Phycomycoses

1. The cerebrorhinoorbital phycomycoses are caused by members of the genera *Absidia, Mucor, Rhizopus,* and *Mortierella.*

2. Most infections occur following a paranasal sinus infection in diabetics in acidosis, and in other immunocompromised hosts.

3. The fungi invade blood vessels and often cause death within a week.

4. Amphotericin B and 5-flucytosine are the drugs of choice.

Protozoal Infections

1. Some trypanosomes, toxoplasmas, and amebas can penetrate the cribriform plate or reach the meninges.

2. The brain and meninges may be involved in amebic meningoencephalitis, in disseminated toxoplasmosis, and in chronic stages of African sleeping sickness.

3. In some instances, granulomatous lesions that contain the parasites occur in the brain or on the meninges.

4. Some malarial parasites cause brain damage by occluding cerebral capillaries.

Amebic Meningoencephalitis

1. Amebic meningoencephalitis is a rare infection caused by soil amoebas that belong to the genera *Naegleria* or *Acanthamoeba.*

2. The origin of the cysts that can penetrate the cribriform plate is contaminated water.

3. No reliable treatment is available.

Toxoplasmosis

1. Toxoplasmosis is a common infection, but rare disease, that is caused by *Toxoplasma gondii.*

2. Adults are infected by eating raw or inadequately-cooked meat or poultry or by coming in contact with cat feces.

3. Toxoplasmosis can also be transmitted to the fetus by crossing the placenta or during delivery.

4. The protozoan multiplies and encysts in the retina of adults.

5. The amount of damage to a fetus is related to the trimester in which the fetus acquires the disease.

6. The drugs of choice are pyrimethamine and sulfadiazine.

African Sleeping Sickness

1. African sleeping sickness is caused by the hemoflagellate *Trypanosoma brucei gambiense* or *T. b. rhodesiense.*

2. The trypanosomes are transmitted by the bite of a tsetse fly from the genus *Glossina.*

3. Invasion of the central nervous system causes irritability, mental disturbances, and a coma that may last for months or years.

4. Suramin, pentamidine, and melarsoprol are the drugs of choice.

Viral Infections

1. Certain viruses may have an affinity for the central nervous system.

2. Some peripheral nerves house viruses, without apparent effect.

Aseptic Meningitis

1. Aseptic meningitis is an inflammation of the meninges that is assumed to be caused by a virus.

2. Enteroviruses are the most common cause of aseptic meningitis.

3. Most people infected with aseptic meningitis recover without incident in two weeks.

4. There is no specific treatment for aseptic meningitis other than supportive care.

Poliomyelitis

1. Since the development and use of the Salk vaccine in 1955, poliomyelitis has not been a public health problem in the United States.

2. Poliomyelitis is an acute inflammation of the spinal cord and brain stem.

3. Type 1 poliovirus is the most frequent cause of paralytic illness.

4. Most infections are inapparent, and less than 1 percent of symptomatic individuals develop paralysis.

5. No drugs affect the course of paralysis, but poliomyelitis can be prevented by administration of an inactivated poliovirus vaccine (IPV) or a live oral poliovirus vaccine (OPV).

Encephalitis

1. Encephalitis is an inflammation of the brain. It is caused by a variety of etiologic agents, including arthropodborne viruses.

2. Western equine encephalitis (WEE) is transmitted by the *Culex* mosquito.

3. Permanent neurologic impairment is more common in children than in adults.

4. There is no specific treatment, but supportive care is important.

Rabies

1. Rabies is a type of encephalitis caused by a virus found in infected domestic and wild animals.

2. Rabies is transmitted to humans through a bite, an abrasion, or though virus-laden aerosols.

3. The disease in humans is almost always fatal.

4. Rabies can be prevented by the administration of either human diploid cell vaccine (HDCV) or rabies vaccine absorbed (RVA). Rabies immune globulin (RIG) is given postexposure.

Viral Conjunctivitis and Keratitis

1. Viral conjunctivitis with or without keratitis can be caused by a number of viruses.

2. Some cases are extensions of a primary infection, but others are transmitted by contaminated hands, materials, or instruments.

3. Iodo-deoxyuridine (IDU) and corticosteroids may provide symptomatic relief.

Prion-Associated Diseases

1. Diseases that are caused by prions and identified as protein particle infections have a latency period of months or years.

2. Prion-associated diseases in humans include subacute sclerosing panencephalitis (SSPE), kuru, and Creutzfeldt-Jakob disease (CJD).

3. CJD is similar to bovine spongiform encephalitis (BSE), a neurological disorder in cattle known as "mad cow" disease.

4. No specific treatment is available.

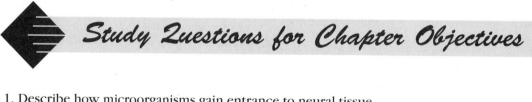

Study Questions for Chapter Objectives

1. Describe how microorganisms gain entrance to neural tissue.

_____

_____

_____

_____

_____

_____

2. List the bacteria that commonly cause meningitis.

_____

_____

_____

_____

3. List the major microbial diseases, and their etiologic agents, for infections of the eye and ear.

_____

_____

_____

_____

_____

4. List the major fungi that cause diseases of the nervous system.

_____

_____

_____

_____

5. List the major protozoa that cause diseases of the nervous system.

_____

_____

_____

_____

6. List the major viral infections of the nervous system.

_____

_____

_____

7. Compare prions and viruses for similarities and differences in nervous system diseases.

_____

_____

_____

_____

_____

8. Explain the significance of the blood-brain and cerebrospinal fluid barriers in preventing and treating infections.

_____

_____

_____

_____

_____

9. How do microorganisms gain access to the eyes and ears?

_____

_____

_____

_____

_____

___10. What is the most common cause of meningitis in very young children?
a. *Neisseria meningitidis*
b. *Haemophilus influenzae* type B
c. *Listeria monocytogenes*
d. *Streptococcus pneumoniae*
e. *Staphylococcus aureus*

Match the disease in column B that is associated with each reservoir in column A. You may use a letter more than once.

Column A	Column B
___11. Carrier	a. Rabies
___12. Pigeon droppings	b. Meningococcal meningitis
___13. *Culex* mosquito	c. *Haemophilus influenzae* type B infection
___14. Soil in wound	d. Tetanus
___15. Animal dung	e. Cryptococcosis
___16. Ponds or water	f. Toxoplasmosis
___17. Human skin	g. Amebic encephalitis
___18. Bats	h. Western equine encephalitis
___19. Infected cats	i. Absidia infection
___20. Skunks	j. Polio
___21. Nasopharyngeal discharge	k. Adenovirus infection

Name one etiologic agent for each disease.

22. Amebic meningoencephalitis: _____

23. Otitis media: _____

24. Western equine encephalitis: _____

25. Bacterial meningitis: _____

26. Trachoma: _____

27. Poliomyelitis: _____

28. Pinkeye: _____

29. Rabies: _____

30. Tetanus: _____

31. African sleeping sickness: _____

32. Kuru: _____

33. Viral conjunctivitis: _____

34. Name four possible complications of otitis media. _____

_____

_____

_____

35. What is responsible for the dramatic reduction in cases of poliomyelitis in the United States? _____

_____

36. What factors predispose individuals to the phycomycoses? _____

_____

_____

_____

37. How can tetanus be prevented? _____

_____

_____

Case Study

A 49-year-old man, who lived in a rural area in Missoula County, Montana, went to an emergency room. An antibiotic was prescribed for fever, sore throat, productive cough, and severe right-sided supraorbital pressure and tenderness of several weeks' duration. He returned five days later and showed confusion, ataxia, persistent fever, cough, and sinus pressure. Standard neurologic evaluations and brain CT tests were normal. The next day, the man exhibited ataxia and had decreased sensation in his right hand. Four days later, the patient had multiple seizures followed by coma and loss of brain stem reflexes. Viral encephalitis was presumptively diagnosed, and intravenous acyclovir therapy was initiated. Three days later, specimens were taken to test for rabies. Antibodies for rabies were detected in the serum. The patient was removed from life-support, and he died.

___38. The etiologic agent is from what group?

a. Bacteria
b. Fungi
c. Protozoa
d. Virus
e. None of *a* though *d* choices

___39. The etiologic agent is transmitted by?

a. Infected saliva
b. Bat droppings
c. An animal bite
d. Aerosols that contain viruses
e. All of *a* though *d* choices

___40. The patient lived in a rural area, and his family reported seeing bats flying near their home. The likely source of his infection is?

a. A dog bite
b. Bat droppings or aerosols
c. A skunk bite
d. Contact with a wolf
e. None of *a* though *d* choices

___41. Family and health care workers were treated prophylactically for exposure to the agent by injections of?

a. Human diploid cell vaccine
b. Rabies vaccine adsorbed
c. Rabies immune globulin
d. A combination of vaccine and immune globulin
e. None of *a* though *d* choices

___42. Effective control of this disease is possible in the United States because of?

a. Compulsory vaccination of dogs and cats
b. Registration of dogs
c. Quarantine of animals that bite humans
d. All of *a* though *c* choices
e. None of *a* though *c* choices

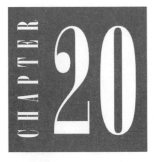

Diseases of the Blood, Lymph, and Immune System

Learning Objectives

1. Explain the role of circulating and sessile cells of the blood and lymph.
2. Compare the life cycles of malarial parasites in mosquitoes and humans.
3. Explain why malaria is still so prevalent in certain parts of the world.
4. Explain the geographic distribution of diseases of the blood, lymph, and immune system.
5. Explain why persons with HIV are so vulnerable to other infectious agents.
6. Discuss the life cycles and geographic distribution of the etiologic agents of Chagas' disease and leishmaniasis.

Study Outline

Introduction

1. Circulating cells of the blood, lymph, and immune system include macrophages, red blood cells, white blood cells, and platelets.
2. The macrophages found in a number of organs are sessile cells such as the Kupffer cells of the liver, osteoclasts of bone, and microglial cells of nerve tissue.
3. Blood and lymph can transport microorganisms far from the point of entry.
4. Some microorganisms escape phagocytic activity and multiply in lymph nodes to produce buboes.

Bacterial Infections

1. In primary bacteremias, bacteria enter the bloodstream through wounds, burns, and bites, or by penetrating the skin.
2. The types of bacteria that gain access to the bloodstream vary with geographic areas and the type of health care available.

3. Positive blood cultures are always significant because blood is normally sterile.

Common Bacteremias

1. Both gram-positive and gram-negative organisms cause bacteremias.
2. Fever is the most frequent sign of sepsis.
3. Isolation of etiologic agents may require at least three blood cultures taken from different sites.
4. Antibiotic susceptibility tests are necessary to determine treatment of choice.

Brucellosis (Undulant Fever)

1. Brucellosis is caused by *Brucella abortus, B. melitensis, B. suis,* or *B. canis.*
2. It is transmitted by contaminated milk or dairy products, infected animals, or the inhalation of aerosols.
3. Fever, headache, and generalized aches often last a long time because *Brucella* organisms persist in macrophages.
4. The drugs of choice are tetracycline and streptomycin.

Plague

1. Plague is a serious disease of the lymph nodes, blood, or lungs.
2. The etiologic agent, *Yersinia pestis,* is transmitted by the rat flea *Xenopsylla cheopis* or by aerosols.
3. Buboes may be present in the inguinal, axillary, or cervical areas.
4. Streptomycin, tetracycline, or chloramphenicol are effective.
5. A vaccine of killed *Y. pestis* cells is available.

Tularemia

1. Tularemia is a disease of the blood and lymph nodes and is caused by *Franciscella tularensis.*
2. It is transmitted by the direct inoculation of skin or mucous membranes, and by ticks, deer flies, and mosquitoes.
3. Infection of the blood and lymph nodes may be followed by lung or gastrointestinal disease.
4. Streptomycin is the drug of choice.
5. A live attenuated vaccine has reduced the incidence of tularemia in laboratory personnel.

Rocky Mountain Spotted Fever

1. Rocky Mountain spotted fever is caused by *Rickettsia rickettsii* and occurs throughout the United States.
2. It is transmitted by the ticks *Dermacentor andersoni* and *D. variabilis.*
3. The multiplication of the rickettsia in the endothelial lining of arterioles and capillaries causes a high fever and rash on the extremities.
4. Tetracycline or chloramphenicol is the drug of choice.

Other Rickettsial Diseases

1. Rickettsial diseases other than Rocky Mountain spotted fever and Q fever are not common in the United States.
2. The infections are transmitted by lice, fleas, mites, or aerosol.
3. A hallmark of miteborne typhus fever is a skin ulcer, known as an eschar, found at the site of mite attachment.
4. Tetracycline or chloramphenicol are effective.

Lyme Disease

1. The spirochete *Borrelia burgdorferi* is transmitted by infected tick bites of the *Ixodes* species.

2. A minimum of a 24-hour attachment by the nymph stage is required for transmission to occur.
3. Neurologic, cardiac, and joint disease are common complications.
4. Treatment involves penicillin or tetracycline.

Ehrlichiosis

1. The etiologic agent of human monocytic infection is *Ehrlichia chafeensis;* of human granulocytic infection, it is *E. equi.*
2. The bacterial agent is transmitted by a tick bite.
3. Tetracycline is recommended in suspected cases.

Relapsing Fever

1. Relapsing fever, a disease characterized by recurrent febrile episodes, is caused by the spirochete *Borrelia recurrentis.*
2. Epidemic relapsing fever is transmitted by the lice *Pediculus humanus corporis* and *P. humanus capitis.*
3. Endemic relapsing fever is transmitted by ticks that belong to the genus *Ornithodoros.*
4. Penicillin, tetracycline, or chloramphenicol are used in the treatment.

Cat-Scratch Disease

1. Cat-scratch disease is a subacute, self-limiting disease that develops after receiving a scratch or bite from a cat.
2. The etiologic agent is the gram-negative bacillus *Bartonella henselae.*
3. Antibiotics do not alter the course of the disease.

Viral Infections

1. Signs and symptoms may not be present in viral infections of the blood until the viruses localize in the liver, spleen, or endothelial cells of capillaries.
2. Most primary viremias are transmitted by arthropod vectors.
3. Life-threatening viral infections are more common in tropical and subtropical climates.

Infectious Mononucleosis

1. This is usually a self-limiting disease of the lymphatic system. It is most often caused by the Epstein-Barr virus (EBV) or the cytomegalovirus (CMV).
2. It is chiefly a disease among young adults who live in developed countries.

3. The association of EBV with Burkitt's lymphoma and nasopharyngeal carcinoma in some parts of the world is not well understood.
4. EBV is transmitted by oral contact, blood, blood products, and bone marrow transplants.
5. A prominent feature of infectious mononucleosis is the presence of atypical lymphocytes.
6. There is no specific treatment for the disease.

Acquired Immunodeficiency Syndrome (AIDS)

1. Human immunodeficiency virus types 1 and 2 (HIV-1 and HIV-2) infect and destroy CD4+ T lymphocytes.
2. AIDS is transmitted sexually, by placental or breast milk transfer, and contact with body fluids.
3. AIDS is a leading cause of death in men and women ages 25 to 44.
4. An ELISA and a Western blot test usually detect the presence of HIV antibodies within three months after exposure to the virus.
5. Drugs to inhibit the action of reverse transcriptase and protease are used to treat HIV infection and AIDS, but do not cure them.

Viral Hemorrhagic Fevers

1. The viral hemorrhagic fevers occur in many parts of the world, but they occur in larger numbers in tropical and subtropical climates.
2. The etiologic agents include members of the arenaviruses, bunyaviruses, flaviviruses, and filoviruses.
3. Yellow fever and dengue are transmitted by the mosquito *Aedes aegypti;* dengue is also transmitted by *A. albopictus.*
4. There is no specific treatment for viral hemorrhagic fevers, but blood transfusions are often required.
5. A vaccine consisting of an attenuated strain of the yellow fever virus is available.

Protozoal Infections

1. All protozoa that infect blood, lymph, or organs of the immune system require an arthropod to complete their life cycle.
2. The parasites are transmitted to humans through the bite of an infected arthropod.

Malaria

1. Malaria is an acute and sometimes chronic disease that affects 300 million people a year.
2. The etiologic agents are *Plasmodium vivax, P. malariae, P. falciparum,* and *P. ovale.*
3. The disease is transmitted by female *Anopheles* mosquitoes and by blood transfusions or contaminated syringes.
4. The human is the intermediate host for the phase of asexual reproduction known as schizogony, which destroys erythrocytes.
5. The phase of sexual reproduction known as sporogony takes place in mosquitoes, the definitive hosts.
6. The asexual phase has an exoerythrocytic and an erythrocytic developmental period.
7. The time required for development of the parasites in the erythrocytes coincides with the periodicity of fevers.
8. Fertilization occurs in the stomach of the mosquito when microgametocytes enter the cytoplasm of macrogametocytes in order to form zygotes.
9. Chloroquine, sulfonamides, and pyrimethamine are used to treat malaria.
10. Development of a vaccine is hampered by the mutability of the parasite's surface antigens.

Babesiosis

1. Babesiosis is a rare but serious disease that occurs primarily in immunocompromised hosts.
2. The etiologic agents are *Babesia microti, B. bigemina,* and perhaps other *Babesia* species.
3. The disease is transmitted by *Ixodes* ticks and carried by deer mice and field mice.
4. Pentamidine reduces the degree of parasitemia in babesiosis.

Chagas' Disease (American Trypanosomiasis)

1. Chagas' disease occurs primarily in children who live in rural central and south America.
2. The etiologic agent *Trypanosoma cruzi* is transmitted by the bite of reduviid bugs that belong to the genus *Triatoma,* by blood transfusions, and by crossing the placental barrier.
3. Epimastigote and trypomastigote developmental forms of the parasite occur in reduviid bugs and in humans.

4. Promastigote and amastigote developmental forms also occur in humans.

5. Rodents and armadillos are reservoirs of the reduviid bugs.

6. The drug of choice is nifurtimox.

Leishmaniasis

1. Visceral leishmaniasis or kala azar is a chronic systemic disease caused by *Leishmania donovani.*

2. Cutaneous leishmaniasis is a localized, less serious infection caused by *L. tropica, L. braziliensis,* or *L. mexicana.*

3. The bite of infected sandflies belonging to the genus *Phlebotomus* transmit the disease.

4. Only the developmental phase known as amastigotes or Leishman-Donovan (LD) bodies occurs in humans.

5. A type of cutaneous leishmaniasis in which ulcerative metastases occurs is known as espundia.

6. Pentavalent antimony is the drug of choice for lesions caused by *L. braziliensis,* and for visceral leishmaniasis.

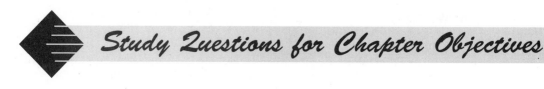

Study Questions for Chapter Objectives

1. List the types and explain the role of circulating and sessile cells of the blood and lymph in infection.

_____

_____

_____

_____

_____

_____

_____

_____

_____

_____

_____

_____

_____

_____

Compare the life cycles of malarial parasites in mosquitoes and humans. Match a letter in column B with an item in column A.

Column A

____2. Definitive host

____3. Intermediate host

____4. Site of schizogony

____5. Site of sporogony

____6. Sexual stages form

____7. Sexual stages fuse

____8. Gametocytes develop in

____9. Sporozoites develop in

___10. Merozoites develop in

___11. Exoerythrocytic period is found in

___12. Erythrocytic period is found in

___13. Ring-form is found in

Column B

a. *Anopheles* mosquito host

b. Human host

c. Both *a* and *b* are correct

d. Neither *a* nor *b* are correct

Fill in the table with the appropriate information.

The names of the species that cause malaria	Erythrocytic Period (Hrs)	Duration of Infection
14.	18.	22.
15.	19.	23.
16.	20.	24.
17.	21.	25.

26. Describe some factors involved in the difficulty with eradication of malaria.

_____

_____

_____

_____

Write the name of a disease transmitted by each vector.

27. *Aedes aegypti:* _____

28. *Xenopsylla cheopis:* _____

29. *Dermacentor andersoni:* _____

30. *Pediculus humanus corporis:* _____

31. *Anopheles* sp.: _____

32. *Triatoma* sp.: _____

33. *Phlebotomus* sp.: _____

34. *Ixodes* sp.: _____

35. *Ornithodoros* sp.: _____

Name one or more etiologic agents for each disease.

36. Brucellosis: _____

37. Visceral leishmaniasis: _____

38. Tularemia: _____

39. Plague: _____

40. Relapsing fever: _____

41. Lyme disease: _____

42. Infectious mononucleosis: _____

43. Malaria: _____

44. Cutaneous leishmaniasis: _____

45. Rocky Mountain spotted fever: _____

46. What preventive measures can you take to prevent exposure to biting insects?

_____

_____

_____

47. Explain the geographic distribution of diseases of the blood, lymph, and immune system.

_____

_____

_____

_____

48. Discuss the life cycles and geographic distribution of the etiologic agents of Chagas' disease and leishmaniasis.

_____

_____

_____

_____

_____

_____

Case Study

A 29-year-old missionary, Mrs. R. became ill while traveling back to the United States from west Africa. She was suffering from fever, malaise, and abdominal discomfort when she arrived in New York. She was immediately hospitalized and began experiencing some bouts of painful urination. The urine was blood-tinged. The patient reported receiving multiple mosquito bites about 12 days before. Examination of initial blood smears revealed the presence of multiple small ring forms in the red blood cells. A second set of blood smears revealed the presence of gametocytes and Maurer's spots in red blood cells.

___49. What disease did Mrs. R. have?

    a. Yellow fever
    b. Malaria
    c. Lyme disease
    d. Rocky Mountain spotted fever
    e. Plague

___50. What genus of insect bit her?

    a. *Anopheles*
    b. *Culex*
    c. *Ixodes*
    d. *Pediculus*
    e. *Dermacentor*

___51. What is the species that caused her symptoms?

    a. *Plasmodium vivax*
    b. *Plasmodium falciparum*
    c. *Plasmodium malariae*
    d. *Plasmodium ovale*
    e. *Borrelia burgdorferi*

___52. The disease is caused by which organism or particle?

    a. Bacteria
    b. Fungus
    c. Protozoa
    d. Virus
    e. Prion

___53. What are possible precautions Mrs. R. could have taken to prevent contracting the disease?

    a. Worn protective clothing
    b. Used mosquito netting protection when she slept
    c. Sprayed insect repellant on her clothes every day
    d. Limited her travels into mosquito areas, or at night, when mosquitoes are active
    e. All of *a* through *d* choices

CONTROL OF MICROORGANISMS

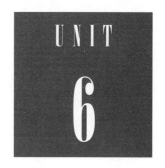

UNIT

6

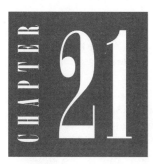

CHAPTER 21

Disinfection and Sterilization

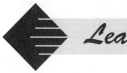

Learning Objectives

1. Differentiate between asepsis, disinfection, sanitation, and sterilization.
2. Describe the factors that influence the death of microorganisms.
3. Contrast the efficiency of the physical agents commonly employed for disinfection and sterilization.
4. Differentiate between thermal death time and thermal death point.
5. Define photoreactivation and photo-oxidation.
6. Classify the major disinfectants as protein-denaturing or membrane-altering agents.
7. Describe two standardized methods for testing the efficiency of disinfectants.

Study Outline

Introduction

1. The process of sterilization destroys all microorganisms.
2. The process of disinfection destroys all pathogenic microorganisms except spores and viruses.
3. Chemical agents that inhibit or kill microorganisms on inanimate objects are disinfectants.
4. Chemical agents that inhibit growth or activity of microorganisms on living tissue are antiseptics.

Factors Influencing Death of Microorganisms

1. The death of microbial populations is affected by the physiological state of the organisms and environmental factors.
2. Microbial susceptibility to biocides is extremely variable.

Size of the Microbial Population

1. The density of large numbers of microorganisms may prevent penetration of an agent.
2. The probability of a direct hit lessens with lower numbers of microorganisms.

Time of Exposure

1. The longer the time of exposure to a lethal agent, the greater is the number of microorganisms killed.

2. Cells of a microbial population are not equally susceptible to antimicrobial action.

Intensity or Concentration of Antimicrobial Agent

1. The destructive power of most disinfectants increases exponentially with increasing concentration up to an optimum concentration.

2. Each chemical agent has an optimal microbicidal concentration for an application.

Type and Age of Microorganisms

1. Some fungi and viruses are more resistant to physical and chemical agents than vegetative cells of bacteria.

2. Staphylococci, enterococci, and some gram-negative bacteria are quite resistant to disinfectants.

3. The hydrophobic nature of cell surfaces of mycobacteria provides some protection from the lethal effects of aqueous chemical agents.

4. Cells in the exponential growth phase are the most susceptible to heat.

5. The vulnerability of spores to physical and chemical agents is related to age of the spores and environmental factors present during their formation.

Properties of Contaminated Materials

1. Plastic, rubber, or instruments with fine cutting edges cannot withstand moist heat or corrosive chemicals.

2. Some chemical agents destroy delicate fabrics.

3. Viscous contaminated fluids or the presence of extraneous organic materials require greater exposure time or increased concentration of disinfectant to destroy microorganisms.

Environmental Conditions

1. An increase in temperature usually enhances the destructive ability of disinfectants.

2. The synergistic effect of heat, oxygen, and an acid pH often lowers the time of exposure to an antimicrobial agent required for disinfection or sterilization.

Physical Agents

1. When the nature of the contamination is known, the appropriate physical limitation can be applied effectively.

2. More stringent methods of decontamination must be applied if the nature of the contaminant is not known.

Heat

1. Dry heat, moist heat, or steam under pressure can be used to destroy microorganisms.

2. Dry heat causes oxidation of cell substances whereas moist heat, with or without pressure, causes coagulation of cell proteins.

3. Some viruses are inactivated at room temperature, but others are destroyed only after prolonged exposure to heat.

4. Thermal death time is the length of time required to kill a particular organism at a specific temperature.

5. Thermal death point is the temperature required to kill a particular micro-organism within 10 minutes.

Dry Heat

1. Incineration and flaming are efficient uses of dry heat for certain disposable materials or for objects which can withstand intense heat.

2. Exposure to temperatures of 160 to 180°C for two hours or longer is necessary to sterilize glassware.

Moist Heat

1. Moist heat can accomplish sterilization at lower temperatures and shorter times of exposure than dry heat.

2. Vegetative cells of bacteria can be destroyed by boiling for 20 minutes.

3. Tyndallization requires a 30-minute exposure to steam on three successive days to kill sporeformers.

4. Steam under pressure in an autoclave is the most efficient method of sterilization with 15 pounds of pressure per square inch raising steam temperature to 121°C for sterilization.

Cold

1. Low temperatures inhibit the growth of most microorganisms, but do not kill most organisms.

2. Osmotic pressure, pH, and humidity influence destruction of microorganisms at low temperatures.

Desiccation

1. Most microorganisms can survive in an environment of low moisture content.
2. Lyophilization (rapid freezing and drying) is used to preserve some biological products.
3. Stock bacteriological and tissue cultures are often stored under liquid nitrogen at -196°C.

Osmotic Pressure

1. Most microorganisms do not tolerate an environment in which the external concentration of solute exceeds that of cells.
2. Osmotic tolerance is expressed in terms of lowest water activity (a_w) permitting growth.

Filtration

1. Membrane filtration can remove all microorganisms including some viruses from liquids and air.
2. Membrane filters of cellulose acetate or cellulose nitrate have wide application in industrial and hospital laboratories.

Radiation

1. Radiation consists of the propagation of energy through space as electromagnetic waves.
2. Wavelength of electromagnetic waves is usually expressed in nanometers (nm).

Ultraviolet

1. Ultraviolet radiation (UV) causes the formation of thymine dimer bonds in DNA preventing replication of DNA.
2. Some microorganisms are able to repair UV damage of DNA by photo-reactivation enzymes that operate in the presence of light, or by enzymes that promote repair of DNA in the dark.

Visible Light

1. Prolonged exposure of microorganisms to visible light destroys microorganisms by photooxidation.
2. The destructive action of light depends on absorption of light in the absence of oxygen or by the toxic effect of singlet oxygen (O_2^-).
3. Some microorganisms contain protective carotenoid pigments which prevent light from reaching the vulnerable molecules.

Ionizing Radiation

1. The emissions of X-rays, gamma rays, and cosmic rays are highly microbicidal.
2. Ionizing radiation is used to sterilize heat-sensitive items, such as sutures and disposable plastic items.

Microwave Radiation

1. Microwaves have wavelengths between the infrared and radio wave portions of the electromagnetic spectrum.
2. Microwave radiation is not an effective means of decontamination of most materials, but may be useful to sterilize household sponges, dishcloths, and wooden cutting boards.

Chemical Agents

1. Some chemical agents are reliable for disinfection, but not for sterilization.
2. The choice of an appropriate chemical agent depends on the type of material and amount and type of organisms present.
3. The three levels of disinfection are high, intermediate, low.

Protein-Denaturing Agents

1. Microbial cells are vulnerable to chemical agents that change or denature the protein molecules.
2. Some chemical agents alter catalytic sites in enzyme molecules.

Organic Solvents

1. Organic solvents denature proteins and alter permeability of cell membranes.
2. The alcohols are generally safe and inexpensive, but limited in action against spores and viruses.
3. Other solvents are highly germicidal, but may have irritating and carcinogenic properties.

Heavy Metal Compounds

1. Silver, mercury, copper, arsenic, zinc, and others are good disinfectants, but not reliable as biocides.
2. Soluble salts of heavy metals inactivate proteins containing sulfhydryl (SH) groups.

Oxidizing Agents

1. Chlorine, bromine, and iodine solutions have a high degree of germicidal activity.
2. These agents oxidize sulfhydryl groups (SH) and react with amino groups (NH_2) of proteins.

3. Hypochlorites and chloramines are widely used in the treatment of water supplies.

4. Iodine preparations are effective skin disinfectants.

5. Organic bromides are used in hot tubs.

6. Oxygen released from hydrogen peroxide has a toxic effect on anaerobic bacteria that cause wound infections.

Dyes

1. Basic dyes are more effective bacterio-static agents than acidic dyes.

2. Basic dyes such as crystal violet and brilliant green selectively inhibit some gram-positive bacteria.

Alkylating Agents

1. Formaldehyde, glutaraldehyde, and ethylene oxide alter amino (NH_2), hydroxyl (OH), sulfhydryl (SH), and carboxyl (COOH) groups of proteins or nucleic acids.

2. Formalin, an aqueous solution of 5 to 37 percent formaldehyde, is active against vegetative cells and spores.

3. A 2 percent solution of glutaraldehyde disinfects respiratory therapy equipment.

4. Ethylene oxide gas in a sterilizer is used for heat-sensitive materials.

Membrane-Altering Agents

1. Metabolic processes of microbial cells are dependent on the integrity of cell membranes.

2. A change in membrane permeability or structural damage causes a loss of metabolites and provides a portal of entry for harmful agents.

Surface-Active Agents

1. Surface-active agents or detergents are usually used with other disinfectants or soaps, and a mechanical cleansing process is used to scrub the object to be cleaned.

2. The cationic detergents alter the charges on phospholipids of cell membranes.

3. The quaternary ammonium salts (quats) are cationic detergents that are effective on gram-positive bacteria but have limited action on gram-negative bacteria.

Phenolic Derivatives

1. Phenol and its derivatives disrupt cell membranes even in low concentrations.

2. Phenol no longer has general application in hospitals, but cresols or chlorhexidine are often used as disinfectants in house-holds or hospitals.

Evaluation of Disinfectants

1. The efficiency of germicidal activity of a disinfectant is often expressed as the phenol coefficient: the ratio of the highest dilution of a disinfectant that kills in 10 minutes compared to the highest dilution of phenol that kills in 10 minutes.

2. A use-dilution test is a more definitive method for evaluating the efficiency of various dilutions of a disinfectant for killing the test organism on the surface of 10 carriers in 10 minutes.

 Study Questions for Chapter Objectives

1. Define asepsis. _____

_____

_____

2. Define disinfection. _____

_____

_____

3.   Define sanitation._____

_____

_____

4.   Define sterilization. _____

_____

_____

5.   List and describe six factors that influence death of microorganisms.

_____

_____

_____

_____

_____

_____

_____

Match the disinfectants in column A with a mode of action in column B.

Column A

_____6. Household bleach
_____7. 70 percent ethyl alcohol
_____8. Tincture of iodine
_____9. Phenol
_____10. Quaternary ammonium compound
_____11. Glutaraldehyde
_____12. Silver nitrate
_____13. Hydrogen peroxide
_____14. Hexachlorophene
_____15. Bichloride of mercury
_____16. Chlorhexidine
_____17. Hypochlorous acid
_____18. Soaps
_____19. Iodophors
_____20. Ethylene oxide

Column B

a. Denatures protein
b. Alters membrane permeability

21.   Why is it necessary to flame a bacteriological loop before and after inoculating _____

culture media? _____

_____

_____

---

22. Differentiate between thermal death time and thermal death point.

_____

_____

_____

_____

Quantitative Relationships

Answer *a* if *a* is larger or of greater magnitude than *b*.
Answer *b* if *b* is larger or of greater magnitude than *a*.
Answer *c* if both are about the same or if neither apply.

___23. More susceptible to biocides:
a. Enveloped viruses
b. Prions

___24. Less susceptible to biocides:
a. Bacterial spores
b. Fungal spores

___25. More resistant to biocides:
a. Trophozoite stage
b. Cyst stage

___26. Shorter time required to disinfect to low numbers:
a. 10^9 bacterial cells per square millimeter of floor space
b. 10^6 bacterial cells per square millimeter of floor space

___27. Generally more susceptible to heat:
a. Bacterial cells in the logarithmic growth phase
b. Bacterial cells in the stationary growth phase

___28. In general, the destructive ability of a disinfectant increases with:
a. Heat
b. Cold

___29. Lower time of exposure to an antimicrobial agent is required:
a. Synergistic effects of heat, oxygen, and acid pH
b. Increased heat

___30. For some disinfectants, effectiveness depends on:
a. Absence of organic material on a surface
b. Viscosity of the contaminated solution

31. Define photoreactivation and describe the conditions in which it operates.

_____

_____

_____

_____

_____

_____

32.　Define dark repair and describe the conditions in which it operates.

_____

_____

_____

_____

_____

33.　Define photo-oxidation.

_____

_____

_____

_____

Match a letter from column A with an item in column B.

Column A	**Column B**
___34. A disinfectant is compared to phenol	a. Phenol coefficient
___35. *S. typhi* is a test organism	b. Use-dilution test
___36. Antibiotics are tested	c. Both procedures
___37. Disinfectants are tested	d. Neither procedure
___38. *S. aureus* is a test organism	

___39. Report the ratio of highest dilution of compound to highest
　　　 dilution of phenol that kills test organism in 10 minutes

___40. Use-dilution is the reported value

___41. Stainless steel cylinders are swabbed with test organism

___42. Determines the lowest concentration of chemical that kills in 10 minutes

___43. Tested in replicates of ten

Use the graph on the following page showing the action of chemical disinfectants on a surface to answer the questions from this answer key.
　　　 a. Compound X
　　　 b. Compound Y

___44. Which compound acts in the shortest time to reduce the concentration of microorganisms from 10^5 to 10^2?

___45. Which compound reduces the population to 0.5 organisms per ml in less than 10 minutes?

___46. Which compound reduces the population to 0.5 organisms per ml in less than 25 minutes?

___47. Which compound requires a longer time of contact to reduce the organisms to less than one per hundred?

Graph for questions 44 through 47.

The horizontal line marks the point of reduction of the original population of bacteria to a theoretical one-half organism per milliliter.

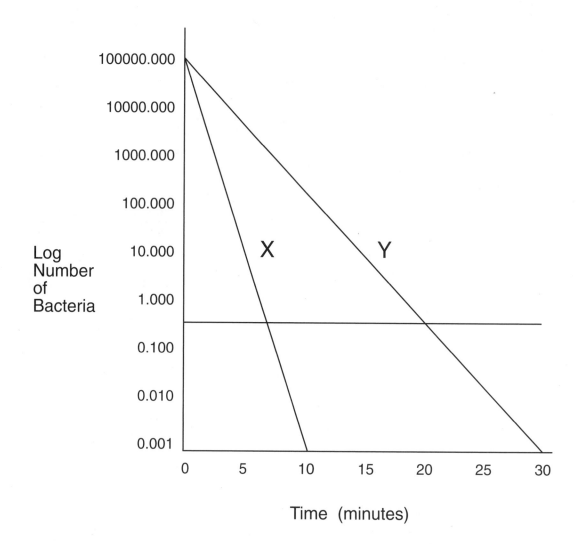

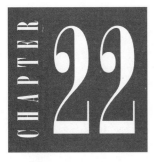

CHAPTER 22

Antimicrobial and Chemotherapeutic Agents

Learning Objectives

1. Distinguish among natural, semisynthetic, and synthetic antimicrobial agents.
2. List the target sites for the major antimicrobial agents.
3. Explain the significance of β-lactamases in the choice of treatment for some infectious diseases.
4. Describe three methods of antimicrobial susceptibility testing.
5. Differentiate between the minimum inhibitory concentration (MIC) and the minimum bactericidal concentration (MBC) of an antibiotic.
6. Describe mechanisms in microorganisms that can lead to developing resistance to antimicrobial drugs.

Study Outline

Introduction

1. The early antibiotics, derived from molds or bacteria, are called natural products, but if they are chemically modified, they are called semi-synthetic.
2. Most antibiotics are classified as secondary metabolites and nonessential for the growth of the producing organism.

Classification of Antimicrobial Agents

1. Antimicrobial drugs exert a microbicidal or a microbiostatic effect on infectious agents.
2. Products that affect only a few types of microorganisms have a narrow-spectrum of activity; products that affect many types of microorganisms have a broad-spectrum of activity.
3. The drugs may be grouped according to the target site of interfering activity.

Antimicrobials Affecting Proteins of Cell Walls and Membranes

1. Penicillins and cephalosporins inhibit synthesis of peptidoglycan molecules, trigger autolytic enzymes, and bind to proteins essential for cell growth.
2. Cycloserine inhibits formation of D-alanine required in synthesis of peptidoglycan molecules.
3. Penicillin and cephalosporin drugs are inactivated by β-lactamases produced by resistant microorganisms, but newer drugs are stable in the presence of ß-lactamases.

Antimicrobials Affecting Lipids of Plasma Membranes

1. Polymyxins and polyenes bind to phospholipid or sterol components of membranes causing leakage of cell contents.
2. Polymyxin B and colistin are bactericidal for gram-negative bacteria, but are limited to use on superficial infections.

3. Amphotericin B, nystatin, candicidin, and the imidazoles are antifungal agents.

Antimicrobials Affecting Protein Synthesis

1. Chloramphenicol blocks the attachment of mRNA to the ribosome; it is not recommended for minor infections.
2. Tetracyclines prevent binding of amino acid-tRNA to the ribosome; side effects include gastrointestinal distress and photosensitivity.
3. The aminoglycosides, such as streptomycin, cause misreading of mRNA resulting in a defective or missing protein.

Antimicrobials Affecting Synthesis of Nucleic Acids

1. Nalidixic acid and related quinolone drugs are potent inhibitors of DNA synthesis by blocking DNA gyrase action; they are active against gram-negative bacteria.
2. The antituberculosis agents, rifampin and rifabutin, block the action of nucleic acid polymerases.
3. Flucytosine is converted to 5-fluorouracil, a base analog of uracil, by fungal enzymes; it is used to treat some fungal infections.

Antimicrobials Affecting Synthesis of Essential Metabolites

1. The sulfonamides competitively inhibit the synthetase enzyme, a first step in the synthesis of folic acid.
2. Trimethoprim, chloroguanide, and pyrimethamine competitively inhibit the reductase enzyme in the synthesis of folic acid.
3. A synergistic effect of sulfonamide with trimethoprim produces as much as a tenfold increase in bacteriostatic activity.
4. Isoniazid interferes with the synthesis of mycolic acid; it is often used with rifampin in the treatment of tuberculosis.

Antimicrobials Having Lesser Known Mechanisms of Action

1. Quinine and its derivatives chloroquine and primaquine are used to treat and prevent malaria, but some strains of *Plasmodium falciparum* are resistant to more than one drug.
2. Chloroquine interferes with activity of malarian parasites in erythrocytes, but primaquine eliminates extra-erythrocytic stages.
3. Metronidazole is an amebicide that is also effective against *Trichomonas vaginalis.*

4. Atovaquone interferes with electron transport in *Plasmodium* species, and inhibits *Pneumocystis carinii* by an unknown mechanism of action.
5. Griseofulvin is effective in treating skin infections by fungi.

Laboratory Methods

1. The goal of drug therapy in infections or neoplastic disease is to provide the most effective treatment with minimum risk and cost to the patient.
2. Laboratories can identify etiologic agents, determine antimicrobial susceptibilities, and monitor levels of antibiotics in the patient's serum.

Antimicrobial Susceptibility Tests

1. If the antimicrobial susceptibility of an etiologic agent is not known or unpredictable, susceptibility testing provides a reliable guide for treatment.
2. Tests should be performed on pure cultures obtained from the patient.

The Kirby-Bauer Method

1. The Kirby-Bauer method employs disks containing antimicrobial agents, and standardized suspensions of bacterial isolates on agar.
2. The diameter of the clear zone of inhibition around each disk is measured in millimeters, and interpreted as either susceptible (S), intermediate (I), or resistant (R).

Minimum Inhibitory Concentration and Minimum Bactericidal Concentration

1. Serial twofold dilutions of antibiotics are made in tubes or wells containing broth and a standardized bacterial inoculum.
2. After overnight incubation the lowest concentration of antimicrobials inhibiting visible growth is reported as the minimum inhibitory concentration (MIC).
3. The minimum bactericidal concentration (MBC) is the lowest concentration of an antibiotic that kills the organism measured by subculturing the clear broths of an MIC test onto agar; the failure to produce colonies is the measure of killing.

Rapid Detection of β–Lactamase Activity

1. Production of β-lactamase by bacteria can be detected rapidly using a moistened nitrocefin disk; a positive result confirms resistance of the microorganism to penicillin, ampicillin, and amoxicillin.

2. A cefoxitin disk induction test detects inducible β-lactamase.

Resistance to Antimicrobial Agents

1. Widescale use and abuse of antimicrobial agents selects for the survival of resistant organisms.
2. Changes in patient and physician behaviors are very important in reducing the survival of drug-resistant strains.

Mechanisms of Microbial Resistance

1. Resistance arises from mutations or by gene transfer.
2. A single gene resistance may lead to multiple drug resistance.
3. Mechanisms of resistance to antimicrobial agents that may be developed by a microorganism include blocking entry of an antibiotic into the cell, altering cell targets so they are not vulnerable to drug action, inactivating drugs, and making alternate enzymes that bypass a pathway blocked by drug action.

 Study Questions for Chapter Objectives

Select from the *a* through *e* choices below for questions 1 to 5:
  a. Semisynthetic
  b. Synthetic
  c. Narrow-spectrum
  d. Broad-spectrum
  e. Natural

____1. Antibiotics with a range of activity limited to one type or group of organism
____2. Antibiotics derived from natural sources and modified partially by chemical procedures
____3. Antibiotics with a range of activity against a large number of types or groups of organisms
____4. Antibiotics derived from natural sources
____5. Antibiotics derived from chemical procedures completely

Identify the target site in column B for each antimicrobial agent listed in column A.

Column A	Column B
____6. Penicillin	a. Cell wall and membrane proteins
____7. Nystatin	b. Membrane lipids
____8. Chloramphenicol	c. Protein synthesis
____9. Tetracyclines	d. Nucleic acid synthesis
___10. Streptomycin	e. Synthesis of essential metabolites
___11. Sulfonamides	
___12. Cephalosporin	
___13. Ribavirin	
___14. Isoniazid	
___15. Amphotericin B	
___16. Erythromycin	
___17. Ampicillin	
___18. Azithromycin	
___19. Rifampin	
___20. Zidovudine	

21. Explain the significance of β-lactamases in the choice of treatment for some infectious diseases.

_____

_____

_____

_____

_____

_____

The following results were obtained with ampicillin on strains of *Escherichia coli* (A), *Staphylococcus aureus* (B), and *Haemophilus influenzae* (C) in the Kirby-Bauer testing method. Examine Table 22-3 in the textbook to help you answer questions 22 to 25.

Organism	Zone diameter	Lab Report
A	18 mm	S
B	26 mm	R
C	18 mm	R

22. How can you explain that the zone for organism B was largest and yet was reported resistant?

_____

_____

_____

23. Why must antimicrobial susceptibility tests be performed on pure cultures?

_____

_____

_____

24. Explain why the zone for organism C was the same as the zone for organism A and they were not both reported as susceptible.

_____

_____

_____

25. Explain how the laboratory determines the value of S, R, and I in the interpretation of susceptibility test results.

_____

_____

_____

_____

Identify the type of antimicrobial test in column B with the statement in column A. A letter may be used more than once.

Column A
____26. Uses Mueller-Hinton agar and paper disks.
____27. Uses broth tubes with varying dilutions of antimicrobial agent.
____28. Uses an agar plate inoculated with samples from a clear broth containing a dilution of antimicrobial and an inoculated organism.
____29. Antibiotics are contained on paper disks.
____30. Results are based on looking for no growth in tubes.
____31. Results are based on measuring zone diameters around disks.
____32. Measures the bacteriocidal level of an antimicrobial agent.
____33. Measures the concentration of antimicrobial agent that inhibits or kills a bacterium.
____34. Results are reported as R, S, or I.
____35. Reported as a concentration that kills a bacterium.
____36. Reported as the concentration that inhibits visible growth.
____37. Useful for determining appropriate therapy for a patient.
____38. Serial twofold dilutions of an antimicrobial agent are placed in tubes or wells of plastic plates.
____39. The results of these two tests may indicate the same concentration of antimicrobial agent.
____40. Results are necessary for patients with lowered immune responses.

Column B
a. MIC
b. MBC
c. Kirby-Bauer
d. All of *a* through *c* choices
e. Both *a* and *b* choices

41. Describe three human behaviors that may contribute to the emergence of drug-resistant strains of microorganisms.

_____

_____

_____

_____

_____

_____

_____

42. Describe three mechanisms by which microorganisms acquire resistance to anti-microbial agents.

_____

_____

_____

_____

_____

_____

_____

_____

_____

ENVIRONMENTAL AND FOOD MICROBIOLOGY

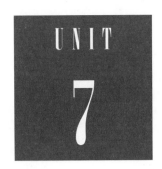

UNIT 7

23 Microbiology of the Environment

Learning Objectives

1. Describe three types of symbiotic relationships involving microorganisms.
2. List specific roles of microorganisms in recycling carbon, nitrogen, and sulfur.
3. Name three major methods used by cities to purify drinking water.
4. Describe methods used in the microbiological examination of water.
5. Describe preliminary, primary, secondary, and tertiary treatments of sewage.
6. Discuss the consequences of human intervention in ecosystems.

Study Outline

Ecosystems

1. Ecosystems consist of biotic and abiotic components of local environments; ecology is the study of biotic and abiotic factors within ecosystems.
2. The physical and chemical properties of ecosystems influence the types and numbers of microorganisms present.

Interactions Among Populations of Organisms

1. A close association between two organisms in a niche is called symbiosis.
2. Symbiotic relationships may be beneficial or harmful to organisms.

Mutualism

1. Each organism benefits from the symbiotic relationship in mutualism.
2. Lichens are prime examples of mutualism between an alga or a cyanobacterium and a fungus.

Commensalism

1. One partner benefits and the other is unaffected in commensalism.
2. Microorganisms on the surface of human skin usually live as commensals on their host.

Parasitism

1. One partner is harmed in parasitism.

2. A parasite feeds on tissue or products of its host and may destroy the host.

The Food Chain

1. Most species of an ecosystem are not symbionts.

2. Each species is part of a food chain and also part of other food chains forming a vast interconnecting food web.

Energy Flow in Ecosystems

1. Sunlight is the major source of energy that is converted to chemical energy by photosynthetic plants and microorganisms.

2. The organisms of an ecosystem consist of producers, consumers, and decomposers.

3. Energy flows through an ecosystem as consumers feed on producers or other consumers; some energy is lost as heat energy and between trophic levels of food chains.

4. Vascular plants, algae, and cyanobacteria are the primary producers on land; vent bacteria may be the primary producers at the ocean depths.

5. Consumers are classified as herbivores (plant eaters), carnivores (animal eaters) or omnivores (plant and animal eaters).

6. The major decomposers are fungi, bacteria, some arthropods, and earthworms.

Biogeochemical Cycles

1. All forms of life require water, a source of energy, and some basic chemical elements.

2. Microorganisms play major roles in biogeochemical cycles.

The Water Cycle

1. Water enters the atmosphere by evaporation from lakes, rivers, and oceans and by transpiration from plants.

2. Atmospheric water returns to land as rain, snow, or hail and penetrates the land or runs across the surface into rivers and oceans.

The Oxygen Cycle

1. Gaseous oxygen (O_2) is released by photosynthetic organisms into the atmosphere.

2. Oxygen is acquired from the atmosphere by aerobic organisms for respiration.

The Carbon Cycle

1. Carbon dioxide (CO_2) is used by photo- or chemosynthetic organisms to make carbon-containing molecules.

2. Aerobic organisms expel CO_2 during respiration.

3. Decomposers digest the complex carbon-containing molecules of dead consumers.

The Nitrogen Cycle

1. Most forms of life cannot use nitrogen gas (N_2) which constitutes approximately 80 percent of the atmosphere.

2. The chemical bonds of atmospheric N_2 are broken by volcanic activity, lightning, and some bacteria.

3. Microorganisms are essential for the nitrogen cycle.

Nitrogen Fixation

1. N_2 may be converted into ammonia (NH_3) or nitrate (NO_3^-) by bacteria.

2. Many different organisms fix nitrogen independently, but species of *Rhizobium* and *Frankia* establish symbiotic relationships with plants to convert nitrogen gas to nitrates.

Ammonification

1. Organic materials in animal wastes, dead animals, and dead plants are decomposed to ammonia (NH_3) by soil bacteria and fungi.

2. Urea is a product of decomposition of proteins; it is further decomposed to ammonia and carbon dioxide gases by soil microorganisms.

Nitrification

1. Species of *Nitrosomonas* and *Nitrosococcus* oxidize NH_3 to nitrous acid or nitrite ion (NO_2^-)

2. NO_2^- is converted to nitric acid or nitrate ion (NO_3^-) by *Nitrobacter* species.

3. NO_3^- is a final electron acceptor for some obligate and facultatively anaerobic bacteria; it is used by plants and algae.

Denitrification

1. Excess NO_3^- and NO_2^- are converted to N_2 by denitrifying bacteria.

2. Runoff of NH_3 and NO_2^- into freshwater lakes and rivers causes eutrophication, a situation of high nutrients that promotes rapid growth of algae and bacteria and causes oxygen depletion.

The Sulfur Cycle

1. Microorganisms reduce or oxidize elemental sulfur (S) or sulfur compounds.

2. Sulfur is required in the synthesis of the amino acids methionine, cystine, and cysteine.

Anaerobic Sulfur Reduction and Oxidation

1. The reduction of SO_4^{2-} to hydrogen sulfide (H_2S) by anaerobic microorganisms occurs in the bottom sediments of bodies of water.

2. Photosynthetic green and purple bacteria oxidize H_2S to elemental sulfur (S) under anaerobic conditions.

Aerobic Sulfur Oxidation

1. Sulfur (S) is rapidly oxidized to SO_4^{2-} under aerobic conditions by *Thiobacillus* and other bacterial species.

2. The sulfates are metabolized by microorganisms or H_2S is excreted.

Cycles of Other Elements

1. Microorganisms are responsible for recycling phosphorus and iron.

2. Complete conversions from organic to inorganic molecules is a cooperative effort of a community of organisms.

Terrestrial Environments

1. Soil is the product of physical, chemical, and biologic processes occurring over hundreds of years.

2. Soil is divided into horizons called A, B, C, and D.

Microbial Populations of Soil

1. Microbial populations of soil reflect available moisture, nutrients, temperature, pH, and degree of aeration.

2. Bacteria are the most abundant microorganisms of soil.

3. A variety of arthropods, insects, and nematodes react with each other and with microbial residents of soil.

Aquatic Environments

1. Water covers at least 70 percent of the Earth's surface.

2. Microbial populations are abundant on the surface and in the sediments of large bodies of water.

Freshwater Environments

1. The physical and chemical characteristics of freshwater influence microbial populations.

2. Temperatures range from 0°C to more than 80°C and pH varies from two to nine; growth of producers is limited to the surface or photic zone.

3. The four zones from the surface to the bottom of lakes and ponds are littoral, limnetic, profundal, and benthic.

4. Microbial populations of rivers and streams are a reflection of surrounding land use; industrial and agricultural wastes are common pollutants.

Marine Environments

1. Ill-defined geographic boundaries and intermixing of ocean waters contribute to the complexity of marine environments.

2. Temperatures of ocean water are progressively lower with depth except in the region of hydrothermal vents.

3. Ocean waters contain dissolved salt concentration of 3.3 to 3.7 percent and range in pH from 6.5 to 8.3.

4. Hydrostatic pressure increases about 1 atmosphere for every 100 meters of depth.

5. Most biologic activity occurs in the photic zone.

6. Hydrothermal fluids are released from hot springs on the ocean floor at temperatures up to 380°C.

7. The thermal vent areas contain at least 300 species of invertebrates and chemoautotrophic bacteria that provide carbon products for the invertebrates.

8. Water of estuaries reflects the quantity and quality of the fresh and salt water they receive and the land use of the surrounding areas.

9. Many marine animals spend the early part of their lives in estuaries.

10. Enteric bacteria and fungi thrive in nutrient-rich estuaries.

Drinking Water

1. Drinking water is obtained by treating the raw water from rivers, streams, lakes, springs, or wells.

2. Potable water meets standards of quality designated by the United States Public Health Service for human consumption.

Methods of Water Purification

1. Three major methods used by cities to make water safe for drinking are sedimentation, filtration, and chlorination.

2. A final chlorine level of 0.2 to 0.6 parts per million (ppm) is safe for consumption.

Microbiological Examination of Water

1. One type of indicator organism that is used to indicate evidence of contamination of water with animal wastes is the coliform bacteria.

2. Other suitable indicator organisms are *Enterococcus faecalis* and *Clostridium perfringens.*

Quantitative Water Analysis

1. Numbers of bacteria present per milliliter of water is a measure of general cleanliness.

2. Standard plate counts determine the efficiency of water purification.

Qualitative Water Analysis

1. Qualitative tests used in water analysis detect the presence of coliforms or other indicator organisms.

2. Coliforms include *Escherichia coli*, *Enterobacter aerogenes*, and *Klebsiella pneumoniae.*

3. Two methods to detect the presence of coliforms are the multiple tube fermentation technique and the membrane filter (MF) method.

Membrane Filter Method

1. The MF method is especially suitable for field use.

2. The presence of more than one coliform colony per 100 ml of water indicates that the water may be unsafe for drinking.

Multiple Tube Fermentation Technique

1. The multiple tube fermentation technique is based on lactose fermentation with production of gas by bacteria.

2. More than one tube in 15 fermentation tubes inoculated with varying amounts of a water sample is presumptive evidence for the presence of coliforms.

3. A statistical chart is consulted to convert the number of tubes showing gas bubbles to the MPN value.

4. Positive presumptive tubes are tested further by confirmatory and completed tests to verify the presence of coliforms and a new MPN value is reported.

5. To meet EPA requirements, coliforms are reported as either present or absent.

Safe Disposal of Sewage and Wastewater

1. Steps in treatment of sewage are divided into preliminary, primary, secondary, and tertiary forms of treatment.

2. Raw sewage entering a treatment plant is called an influent; water leaving a treatment plant is called an effluent.

3. Each step in wastewater and sewage treatment is designed to lower the Biochemical Oxygen Demand (BOD) of the water before releasing the treated effluent to the environment.

Preliminary Treatment

1. This is a series of physical processes to remove bulky solid wastes with bar screens and mechanical rakes.

2. Smaller solid items are settled out in a grit chamber.

Primary Treatment

1. This is a physical process operating primarily by gravity to settle finely suspended solids in primary clarifier tanks.

2. Greases and oils float to the top of the clarifier tank and they are collected for removal.

3. Chemical agents are used in advanced primary treatment to remove 50 to 75 percent of suspended solids.

Secondary Treatment

1. Effluents from primary treatment enter trickling filter and/or activated sludge systems.

2. Trickling filters and activated sludge tanks use biological processes that depend on the decomposing activity of aerobic bacteria to reduce the organic content of wastewater thus lowering its BOD.

3. Solid sludge is pumped from primary tanks to anaerobic digester tanks where the organics are decomposed by anaerobic bacteria to CO_2, methane (CH_4) and hydrogen sulfide (H_2S) gases.

Tertiary Treatment

1. Tertiary treatment removes organic and inorganic components remaining in secondary effluents by physical and chemical means.

2. Effluents from tertiary treatment are used primarily for landscape irrigation, groundwater injection, and industrial use.

3. Reverse osmosis procedures remove nitrates and phosphates thus reducing the likelihood that the treated wastewater causes eutrophication in a receiving body of water.

Human Intervention in Ecosystems

1. Saving crops and preventing vectorborne diseases have polluted the environment with toxic chemicals.

2. Microorganisms have not evolved strategies to degrade all materials humans have introduced into the environment.

3. Some chemicals become more concentrated at each trophic level in aquatic food chains.

4. Denuded forests cause soil erosion and loss of plants and animals.

5. The process of using biological agents to eliminate toxic wastes is called bioremediation.

6. Bacterial strains are genetically modified to expand their decomposing capabilities for unusual and toxic chemicals.

 Study Questions for Chapter Objectives

Match the organism in column A with the process in column B for recycling elements.

Column A

____1. *Azotobacter*

____2. *Chlorobium*

____3. *Rhizobium*

____4. *Nitrosomonas*

____5. *Thiobacillus*

____6. Green plants

____7. *Nitrobacter*

____8. Animals

____9. *Clostridium* species

___10. *Frankia*

Column B

a. Nitrification

b. Symbiotic nitrogen fixation

c. Reduction of sulfur

d. Use atmospheric carbon dioxide

e. Nonsymbiotic nitrogen fixation

f. Produce carbon dioxide

g. Oxidation of sulfur

11. Describe three examples of mutualism occurring in nature. _____

_____

_____

_____

_____

_____

_____

12. Define commensalism and name two skin bacteria that are considered commensals.

_____

_____

_____

_____

13. Define parasitism. _____

_____

_____

Match the process in column B with the statement in column A for water purification. More than one letter may be used for some items.

Column A	Column B
___14. Particles are removed by gravity.	a. Chlorination
___15. Removes foul odors and tastes.	b. Sedimentation
___16. Water passes through sand.	c. Filtration
___17. Water is held in tanks for clarification.	
___18. Alum is added to bind to particles.	
___19. Removes up to 99.5 percent of microorganisms and particles.	
___20. Final level of 0.2 to 0.6 ppm is suitable for consumption.	

21. List three to five factors that limit microbial growth in marine environments.

_____

_____

_____

_____

_____

_____

22. Explain why aquatic producers grow only in surface waters.

_____

_____

_____

23. Explain the significance of biomagnification and bioremediation.

_____

_____

_____

_____

24. Explain how hydrothermal vents differ from other marine ecosystems.

_____

_____

_____

_____

_____

Match an item in Column A with an appropriate test for the microbiological examination of water quality in Column B. A letter may be used more than once.

Column A	Column B
___25. Coliforms are indicator organisms.	a. Standard plate count
___26. Colonies are counted on agar.	b. Membrane filter
___27. Gas bubbles are counted.	c. Presumptive test
___28. Statistical table provides results.	d. Completed test
___29. Aerobic colonies are counted.	e. Confirmed test
___30. Used to determine water potability.	f. Multiple tube test
___31. Potable water has no more than 100 colony forming units per ml.	g. All of *a* through *f* choices
___32. Potable water should have <4.5 coliforms per 100 ml of water sample in a 15 tube test.	h. Choices *c*, *d*, *e*, *f*
___33. Lactose fermentation is measured.	
___34. Metallic green colonies on the filter are coliforms.	
___35. Positive confirmed test results may be inoculated into one lactose broth tube and one nutrient agar slant.	
___36. Lauryl tryptose broth or lactose broth is used.	
___37. MPN result is reported.	
___38. Has three parts to testing procedure.	
___39. Microscopic examination of cells in colonies is made.	

Quantitative Relationships

Answer *a* if *a* is larger or of greater magnitude than *b*.

Answer *b* if *b* is larger or of greater magnitude than *a*.

Answer *c* if both are about the same or if neither apply.

___40. The BOD value is greater:
   a. Raw influent
   b. Treated effluent

___41. The BOD value is greater:
   a. Primary clarifier tanks
   b. Activated sludge tanks

___42. Microorganisms are responsible for lowering BOD:
   a. Trickling filter tank
   b. Activated sludge tank

___43. Methane gas is produced in larger quantities:
   a. Activated sludge tank
   b. Anaerobic sludge digester tank

___44. Physical particles and chemicals are lowest:
   a. Secondary treatment
   b. Tertiary treatment

Match a wastewater treatment process in column B with a statement in column A.

Column A

___45. Removal of rocks, grit, bulky items

___46. Produces RO water

___47. Physical removal of fats and sludge

___48. Aerobic microorganisms decompose wastes

___49. Anaerobic microorganisms decompose wastes

___50. Reduces BOD

___51. Physical and chemical processes used on water obtained from trickling filters and activated sludge

Column B

a. Preliminary

b. Primary

c. Secondary

d. Tertiary

e. All of *a* through *d* choices

___52. The preliminary treatment of wastewater includes?
   a. Trickling filter tanks
   b. Bar screens and rakes, grit chambers
   c. Activated sludge tanks
   d. Reverse osmosis filters
   e. Anaerobic sludge digester tanks

___53. The primary treatment of wastewater includes?
   a. Trickling filter tanks
   b. Bar screens
   c. Grit chamber
   d. Clarifier tanks
   e. Rakes

___54. The secondary treatment of wastewater includes?
   a. Physical removal of particles and solids
   b. Physical removal of gases and odors
   c. Physical removal of greases and oils
   d. Action of decomposer microorganisms
   e. Reverse osmosis

55. Explain how human activities interfere with ecosystems.

_____

_____

_____

_____

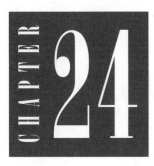

Microbiology of Food and Beverages

Learning Objectives

1. Describe five methods of food preservation.
2. Differentiate between the high-temperature short time (HTST) and the low-temperature long time (LTLT) methods of pasteurization.
3. Explain why heat is more efficient as a food preservative than cold.
4. Describe the two microbiological stages for making vinegar.
5. Name the type of starter cultures and the type of change they produce when used in the production of butter, yogurt, cottage cheese, wine, beer, and bread.
6. Identify microorganisms commonly involved in foodborne illnesses and the types of food generally implicated.

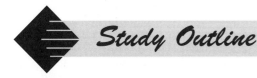
Study Outline

Methods of Food Preservation

1. Food preservation methods have developed over thousands of years in order to provide stabilized foods that do not easily spoil.
2. Modern knowledge of microorganisms, enzymes, and foods allows the choice of an appropriate preserving method.

Heat

1. Nicolas Appert introduced heating of food in sealed containers in 1809 to prevent spoilage.
2. Heating methods can either sterilize canned products or reduce the total number of organisms present.

Dry Heat

1. Any reduction in moisture content of food delays food spoilage.
2. The a_w is a measure of dryness by indicating the water vapor pressure in a food compared to pure water.

Moist Heat

1. Moist heat is a more efficient form of food preservation than dry heat because it uses lower temperatures and shorter times.
2. The high-temperature short time (HTST) method for pasteurization heats milk to a temperature of 71.7°C for 15 seconds.
3. The low-temperature long time (LTLT) method for pasteurization heats milk to a temperature of 62.8°C for 30 minutes.
4. Ultrahigh temperature (UHT) for pasteurization heats milk, fruit juices, fruit, or alcoholic beverages between 140° and 150°C for a few seconds to achieve commercial sterility.
5. Canning of food employs a process of commercial sterilization.
6. The D value is the time required to kill 90 percent of the microorganisms or spores at a certain temperature.

Cold

1. Low temperatures inhibit activity of naturally occurring enzymes and microorganisms in food.
2. Enzymes and some microorganisms are inactivated in vegetables by scalding or blanching before freezing.
3. The keeping quality of refrigerated food is limited and varies with the type of food.
4. Gram-positive bacteria survive better than gram-negative bacteria in frozen foods.

Radiation

1. Ultraviolet light reduces surface contamination, but has limited penetrating power.
2. Low doses of ionizing radiation of x-rays or gamma rays improve keeping qualities of some foods.
3. The dosage of radiation required for sterilization produces undesirable changes in the quality and nutritive value of foods.
4. Microwaving foods destroys microorganisms without other significant changes.

Chemical Agents

1. The FDA allows the addition of approximately 100 chemicals generally regarded as safe (GRAS) to inhibit growth of some microorganisms.
2. Sodium nitrate or nitrite is used in curing meat to inhibit the growth of *Clostridium botulinum*.
3. Sulfur dioxide or sodium sulfite is used to prevent bacterial growth in dried fruits, fruit juices, and wines.

Microorganisms in Food Production

1. The growth of naturally occurring organisms in some foods produces useful products.
2. Starter cultures of bacteria or yeasts are added to some foods to produce desired flavors or textures.
3. The products of fermentation create an unfavorable environment for spoilage microorganisms.

Vinegar

1. Vinegar is made in a two-step process: first, glucose is converted to ethyl alcohol and carbon dioxide by yeasts; second, the alcohol is oxidized to acetic acid.
2. Mixed cultures of acetic acid bacteria, such as *Acetobacter aceti*, are used to generate acetic acid from the alcohol.

Sauerkraut

1. Sauerkraut is a product made from fermentation of shredded cabbage in a salt brine under anaerobic conditions.
2. Naturally occurring lactic acid bacteria produce a final product containing about 1.25 percent lactic acid and other compounds.

Cucumber Pickles

1. Cucumber pickles are often products of complete or limited fermentation in the presence of salt.
2. *Lactobacillus plantarum* is the major producer of the lactic acid fermentation.

Milk Products

1. High quality fermented milk products are obtained by adding starter cultures after pasteurization.
2. The microorganisms of the starter cultures ferment the milk sugar lactose to lactic acid and other compounds.

Butter, Buttermilk, and Sour Cream

1. Butter is made by adding lactic acid and diacetyl-producing bacteria, such as *Streptococcus diacetylactis* or *Leuconostoc citrovorum*, to pasteurized cream.
2. The acidified cream is churned to produce butter.

Yogurt

1. Yogurt is prepared by adding *Streptococcus thermophilus* and *Lactobacillus bulgaricus* to concentrated skim milk.
2. *S. thermophilus* ferments lactose first in the neutral pH of milk to an acidic environment; *L. bulgaricus* ferments lactose in the acidic environment.

Sweet Acidophilus Milk

1. Sweet acidophilus milk is not fermented; it contains low-fat milk and the bacterium, *Lactobacillus acidophilus*.
2. Some persons with gastrointestinal distress following long-term antimicrobial therapy find relief from symptoms if they consume this milk to replace normal intestinal flora killed during therapy.

Cheeses

1. Cottage cheese is made by inoculating whole or skim milk with *Lactococcus lactis* and *Leuconostoc citrovorum*.
2. Ripened cheeses are produced by processes that include curdling milk by the action of enzymes and starter bacteria, removal of whey, salting of curds, and ripening of curds in aging rooms; and for mold-ripened cheese, the addition of fungi.

3. Ripened cheese is classified as soft, semisoft, or hard depending on the water content of the final product.

Bread

1. Strains of *Saccharomyces cerevisiae* are used to make raised bread.
2. Sourdough bread is obtained by adding lactic acid bacteria to the mixture.

Microorganisms in the Production of Alcoholic Beverages

1. Beer making dates back at least 4000 years.
2. Modern production of alcoholic beverages is an applied science.

Wine

1. Winemaking depends on the fermentation of sugars by yeasts to produce ethyl alcohol and carbon dioxide.
2. Wine production begins with the mechanical crushing and pressing of grapes to form a must which is then fermented, clarified, aged, and bottled.
3. Strains of *Saccharomyces ellipsoideus* are used in fermentation.
4. Sparkling wines have a high content of carbon dioxide produced in a secondary fermentation.

Beer

1. Barley or other grains are the source of fermentable sugar in beer making.
2. Strains of *Saccharomyces cerevisiae* or *S. carlsbergensis* are used in the fermentation process.
3. Steps in beer production include malting, kilning, mashing, fermentation of wort with added hops, filtering, and bottling.
4. Light beer is made by pretreating wort with fungal enzymes to reduce the carbohydrate content of the beer.

Microorganisms as a Food Source

1. A high protein product derived from microorganisms is called single-cell protein (SCP).
2. Feeding SCP to livestock could save plant foods for human consumption.
3. The photosynthetic algae *Scenedesmus* and *Spirulina* are sources of SCP.

Transgenic Plants and Animals

1. Genetically modified organisms that have received genes from a different species are known as transgenic plants and animals.
2. Transgenic tomatoes with delayed ripening and improved flavor are available in the U.S.
3. Transgenic animals may become a source of biological products for human use.

Foodborne Illnesses

1. Foodborne illnesses are considered to be either food infections, food poisonings, or a combination of both.
2. Unsanitary food preparation or improper handling of food may introduce pathogenic organisms into food.
3. One of the most common foodborne illnesses is caused by *Staphylococcus aureus* enterotoxin, a heat-stable toxin that induces explosive diarrhea and vomiting.

Microbiological Examination of Foods and Dairy Products

1. Specifications established by regulatory agencies representing the food industry set acceptable limits of numbers or types of microorganisms in foods.
2. Standards set by the U.S. Department of Agriculture and the Food and Drug Administration set limits of numbers and types of microoganisms in foods by law.

Quantitative Methods

1. Numbers of microorganisms are determined by direct microscopic examination or by standard plate counts.
2. The established microbiological standards for each type of food must be met by any food intended for human consumption.

Qualitative Methods

1. The type of microorganisms may be of greater significance than their total numbers.
2. The presence of coliforms is used as an indicator of possible contamination by human or animal wastes, and by implication, with pathogenic organisms.

Dye-Reduction Tests

1. Dye-reduction tests estimate indirectly the number of bacteria in milk as the dye loses color over time.
2. Rapid reduction of dyes to a colorless state by the action of microorganisms indicates a high bacterial count and makes some milk unsuitable for pasteurization.

Enzyme Assay

1. Alkaline phosphatase, an enzyme in raw milk, is inactivated by pasteurization.
2. A positive test for phosphatase in milk indicates that pasteurization has been inadequate or that raw milk has been added to dairy products.

Study Questions for Chapter Objectives

Match a food preservation method from column B with an item in column A. Students may want to refer to appropriate sections in Chapter 21 for additional background information.

Column A

____1. Kills insects in wheat flour
____2. Dehydrates food
____3. Home canning at 121°C
____4. Nonpenetrating radiation
____5. Closed package contains N_2 gas
____6. Radiation causes heat in food
____7. Industrially canned beans
____8. Chemicals added to cake to inhibit molds
____9. Chemical inhibits bacteria in dried fruit
____10. Chemical inhibits *Clostridium botulinum*
____11. Radiation produces undesirable changes in texture, odor
____12. 71.7°C for 15 seconds
____13. 62.8°C for 30 minutes
____14. Kills insects in herbs, spices
____15. Sterilizes milk
____16. Heat milk to 140°C to 150°C for a few seconds
____17. Radiation destroys mold in bread
____18. Sterilizes at 160°C to 180°C for 2 hours
____19. 0°C to 7°C inhibits enzyme action in food
____20. Inhibits mold in cheese

Column B

a. Sodium propionate
b. Hot air oven
c. HTST method
d. Ultraviolet radiation
e. Gamma rays
f. Commercial sterilization
g. Sulfur dioxide
h. UHT method
i. Modified atmosphere package
j. LTLT method
k. Pressure cooker
l. Sodium nitrate, sodium nitrite
m. Pasteurizer
n. Microwave energy
o. Freezing
p. Sodium benzoate
q. Refrigerator

21. Explain why heat is more efficient as a food preservative than cold. _____

_____

_____

_____

_____

_____

Fill in the blanks.

Vinegar production involves a two step process. The first process converts glucose to

22._____ and 23._____ by the action of

24._____. The second process involves the oxidation of

25._____ by the action of 26._____

to produce 27._____, the main flavoring chemical in vinegar.

Match the species in column A that is the starter culture for one or more fermented foods in column B. A letter may be used more than once.

Column A	Column B
___28. *Lactobacillus plantarum*	a. Cottage cheese
___29. *Lactococcus lactis*	b. Cucumber pickles
___30. *Streptococcus thermophilus*	c. Yogurt
___31. *Streptococcus diacetylactis*	d. Vinegar
___32. *Acetobacter aceti*	e. Sauerkraut
___33. *Saccharomyces cerevisiae*	f. Beer
___34. *Leuconostoc* and *Lactobacillus*	g. Bread
___35. *Lactobacillus bulgaricus*	h. Wine
___36. *Leuconostoc citrovorum*	i. Butter
___37. *Penicillium roquefortii*	j. Mold-ripened cheese
___38. *Propionibacterium shermanii*	k. Propionic acid in swiss cheese
___39. *Penicillium camembertii*	
___40. *Saccharomyces ellipsoideus*	

41. Find the bacterial species in the list of names from questions 28 through 40 and write a *B* next to them.

42. Find the yeast species in the list of names from questions 28 through 40 and write a *Y* next to them.

43. Find the mold species in the list of names from questions 28 through 40 and write an *M* next to them.

44. Find the species that produce lactic acid in the food and write *LA* next to the name.

45. Write the names of the species that produce ethyl alcohol and carbon dioxide gas here.

_____

_____

46. Write the name of the species that produces acetic acid here.

_____

47. Write the name of the species that produces diacetyl here.

_____

48. Explain what is meant by the presence of large numbers of coliforms in milk?

_____

49. Explain the relationship of the presence of coliforms in water as studied in Chapter 23 to that in milk.

_____

_____

_____

_____

50. Explain how single-cell protein (SCP) could limit the devastating effects of severe droughts.

_____

_____

_____

_____

_____

Quantitative Relationships

Answer *a* if *a* is larger or of greater magnitude than *b*.
Answer *b* if *b* is larger or of greater magnitude than *a*.
Answer *c* if both are about the same or if neither apply.

___51. Food more involved in *Staphylococcus aureus* food poisoning:

   a. Ham and cheese sandwiches held at room temperature
   b. Custard pie held for 4 hours at room temperature

___52. *Bacillus cereus* foodborne illness is more likely from:

   a. Mashed potatoes and gravy kept warm for 4 hours
   b. Peanut butter

___53. Hepatitis A virus is more likely from:

   a. Unwashed strawberries with soil
   b. Shellfish eaten raw

___54. *Clostridium botulinum* food poisoning is more likely from:

   a. Improperly canned food
   b. Food that is boiled for 20 minutes

___55. *Aspergillus flavus* food poisoning is more likely from:

   a. Peanuts, peanut butter, ham, bacon
   b. Shellfish raw or cooked

___56. *Gonyaulex catenella* food poisoning is more likely from:

   a. Shellfish having saxitoxin
   b. Mashed potatoes and gravy

CHAPTER 1

Answer Key

1. (A) d; (B) E
2. (A) e; (B) D
3. (A) c; (B) C
4. (A) a; (B) B
5. (A) b; (B) A
6. (A) b; (B) F

7. See the section in chapter 1 that discusses the germ theory for their contributions.

8. g	14. a	20. f
9. l	15. d	21. i
10. c	16. a	22. e
11. b	17. j	23. b
12. h	18. b	24. k
13. d	19. b	25. b

26. b	31. a	36. a
27. c	32. b	37. c
28. e	33. b	38. b
29. a	34. a	39. b
30. d	35. b	40. b

41. Structural features of acellular particles are fewer than those found in cells; no metabolism mechanisms; require cellular host for metabolism; viruses, viroids, and prions are acellular.

42. The idea, developed by Aristotle during the Classical Greek period, spread throughout western Europe. The idea of small animals that arise spontaneously was abandoned when Redi's work on maggots became known. When microorganisms were observed in the 1600's, the idea of spontaneous generation became attached to microorganisms. Various experimenters tried to prove and disprove the theory as it applied to bacteria, but Pasteur's swanneck flask experiments finally succeeded. The attempts to disprove the theory of spontaneous generation took a long time because new life forms were seen with the invention of a microscope that showed bacteria and other microorganisms.

43. Your words based on your knowledge of hospitals and medical personnel will be satisfactory.

44. Phagocytic cells surround bacterial cells and other invaders of our body, and then engulf them and digest them.

45. Recognizing the relationships between different types of microorganisms, and arranging the microorganisms in related groups, helps in their identification. Identification is essential to solving the problems of disease, the transmission of disease, and prevention of epidemics.

Answer Key

1. Carbon; 6
2. Nitrogen; 7
3. Oxygen; 8
4. Hydrogen; 1
5. *Cuprum;* copper
6. *Natrium*; sodium
7. K
8 Ca
9. I
10. S
11. P
12. Cl
13 Fe
14. Mg
15. Potassium; *Kalium*
16. Iron; *Ferrum*
17. I, P, and S are named for the first letter in their chemical name; Ca is identified by the first two letters in its chemical name; Cl and Mg are named by the first and third letters in their chemical name. What other chemical elements start with the letter C or M?
18. e
19. e
20. a; b; d
21. a; b; d
22. c

For questions 23-35: I = ionic; C = covalent; H = hydrogen bonds

23. I
24. C
25. C
26. C
27. H
28. C
29. C
30. H
31. H; C for disulfide bonds
32. C
33. C
34. I
35. I

36. e
37. b
38. b
39. c
40. b
41. c
42. c
43. b
44. a
45. d
46. b

For questions 47-50, refer to chapter 2 in the textbook to check your written answer.

51. mRNA: AUG GUA AUC CUC GGG UAA
    tRNA: UAC CAU UAG GAG CCC AUU

For question 52, refer to chapter 2 in the textbook to check your written answer.

53. Industrial and automotive exhaust systems contribute dioxides to the atmosphere. Are there other sources? Acid rain can change the pH in a pond, stream, river, or lake. The animals and plants that live in the water experience a harsher environment, and some species may not grow well. Carbonates act as buffers. Check the textbook for how buffers act with added acid (H+).

CHAPTER **3** # Answer Key

1. b	**12.** g	**23.** e
2. a; c	**13.** g	**24.** d
3. e	**14.** f	**25.** b
4. f	**15.** a; b; c; d; e	**26.** e
5. g	**16.** f	**27.** a
6. f; g	**17.** a; c	**28.** c
7. e	**18.** e	**29.** Purple
8. a; b; c; d	**19.** e	**30.** Red or pink
9. b	**20.** f	**31.** Red
10. a; b; c; d; e	**21.** b	**32.** Blue
11. f	**22.** d	

For questions 33-36, see Table 3-3 in the textbook.

For questions 37-39, see Table 3-4 in the textbook.

40. The application of a single stain to a heat-fixed smear of cells for 30 to 60 seconds

41. The application of more than one stain to a heat-fixed smear of cells

42. A; background

43. B; cell

44. A; background

45. A; background

46. B; cell

47. B; cell

48. B; cell

49. Bacterial cell walls have an excessive number of negative electrical charges that attract the positive charges on basic dye molecules, so the cell is colored. The negative charges on acidic dye molecules are repelled by the negative charges on the bacterial cell wall. This leaves the cell colorless and the background stained.

50. Dark-field

51. Phase-contrast

52. SEM

53. Fluorescence

54. Phase-contrast

55. Phase-contrast

56. TEM

57. Phase-contrast, bright-field

58. DIC

59. Bright-field

60. Fluorescence

61. Thicker walls of gram-positive cells are dehydrated by alcohol, closing pores, and making it more difficult to decolorize the wall, which leaves the cell purple. The outer membrane of gram-negative cells is dissolved by alcohol, and the walls are very thin, which makes them easier to decolorize and then stain by the safranin counterstain.

62. A chemical that increases the binding of dye to cell. Gram's iodine solution is a mordant.

63. 95 percent ethyl alcohol

64. Acid alcohol

65. The stain used after a decolorizer solution to stain decolorized cells

66. Safranin

67. Methylene blue

68. A

69. Bacteria are so small that the light intensity must be adjusted to a lower intensity to reveal their presence. Unstained cells are more easily seen by reducing light intensity. By contrast microscopy, details of thickness or density of cell structures are revealed by the correct level of illumination. Light intensity may be regulated by 1) opening or closing the iris diaphragm, 2) raising the condenser lens toward the stage for brighter light or lowering the condenser for lower illumination, or 3) increasing the illumination from the substage lamp.

70. The decolorization step is critical in the Gram stain. If too much alcohol is used, the gram-positive cells will look pink and be falsely reported as gram-negative. If too little alcohol is used, gram-negative cells will not be decolorized, and they will be falsely reported as gram-positive.

71. Crystal violet; basic carbolfuchsin

72. Less distortion of cells occurs because fixing is not required. Cells are seen against a dark background, and the technique requires only the bright-field microscope commonly found in laboratories.

73. A wet mount preparation that uses a bright-field microscope (see Fig. 3-14 in the textbook) will show cells or particles that seem to bump and jiggle in one place. A phase-contrast microscope and a wet mount of large protozoan cells will demonstrate cytoplasmic streaming.

74. One of the students carried out the decolorization step incorrectly.

75. Many different stains and techniques reveal the cellular structures by their chemistry, their physical nature, and by the techniques used to color them. For example, endospores are resistant to chemicals that enter the interior unless the primary stain is gently heated as it sits on the bacterial smear. Bacterial flagella are thin structures that are easily torn off of cells in the ordinary method used for preparing the smear of cells on a glass slide. The flagellated cells require special procedures to prepare the smear, and a long staining time for dye molecules to build up on the flagella and thicken their dimensions for bright-field microscopy. The Gram and acid fast stains reveal the chemical and physical differences in the cell walls of bacteria.

CHAPTER 4

Answer Key

1. E	**9.** E	**17.** P	**25.** Cell wall
2. P; E	**10.** P	**18.** P	**26.** Flagellum
3. E	**11.** E	**19.** P; E	**27.** Ribosome
4. E	**12.** E	**20.** E	**28.** Plasma
5. P	**13.** E	**21.** E	membrane
6. P	**14.** E	**22.** E	**29.** Pili
7. E	**15.** E	**23.** E	**30.** Cytoplasm
8. E	**16.** E	**24.** P; E	**31.** Nucleoid

32. Capsule
33. Golgi complex
34. Microfilament
35. Nucleus
36. Nucleolus
37. Chloroplast
38. Endoplasmic reticulum
39. Centriole
40. Flagellum
41. Mitochondrion
42. Cytoplasm
43. Chromosome
44. Ribosomes
45. Lysosome
46. Nuclear membrane
47. Vacuole
48. Plasma membrane
49. Cell wall
50. Maintenance of rigid shape; prevents cell disintegration
51. Movement
52. Protein synthesis
53. Site of enzyme activity; transportation of molecules
54. Adherence to surfaces and to other cells
55. Dissolves molecules in its fluid matrix and suspends structures
56. Carries genetic code that contains information for cellular structures and functions
57. Adherence to solid surfaces and to nutrients; prevents phagocytosis

58. g
59. a
60. c
61. e
62. d
63. f
64. b

65. Nucleus
66. Golgi complex
67. Lysosome
68. Mitochondrion
69. Vesicle
70. Vacuole
71. Chloroplast

72. See Table 4-2 and Figure 4-5 in the textbook to form your own answer in a short essay format.

73. Passive transport processes include diffusion, facilitated diffusion, and osmosis. These processes do not require energy expenditure by the cell. Active transport requires an energy expenditure by the cell to concentrate nutrient molecules inside the cell. The energy may come from the bonds of ATP, or from other energy-rich molecules. See the textbook for a description of each of these processes.

74. The lipopolysaccharide layer (LPS) of the outer membrane of gram-negative bacteria has toxic properties when the bacterial cell dies and the LPS is released. The toxin is classified as an endotoxin because it is part of the cell wall, and it is not secreted or released until the cell dies.

75. Resistant

76. Heating canned foods must be done at appropriate temperatures and pressures so that the food texture and quality are not destroyed, but the spores on the vegetables are destroyed. Some spore-forming bacteria can produce toxins in canned foods that are improperly canned. (See the entries for *Clostridium botulinum* in the textbook.)

77. b
78. b
79. c
80. a

CHAPTER 5

Answer Key

1. d	**3.** c	**5.** d	**7.** b
2. b	**4.** a	**6.** a	**8.** c

Mark your answers for 9-12 on the population-growth curve. Check your answer in the textbook.

13. c	**16.** c	**19.** c	**22.** b
14. d	**17.** a	**20.** c	**23.** c
15. a	**18.** d	**21.** a	**24.** b

25. Generation time is the number of minutes between cell divisions.

26. Logarithmic

For questions 27-29, refer to chapter 5 in the textbook for a discussion of streak, pour, and spread-plate techniques.

For questions 30-31, bacteria do not occur in pure culture in nature; they have many natural competitors. Food and other environmental factors are not at optimal levels for long periods.

For questions 32-40, refer to chapter 5 in the textbook for the information. List answers in any order.

41. This organism would require organic carbon molecules, a temperature of 45°C or more, and the absence of oxygen.

42. Refer to chapter 5 in the textbook for a discussion in the section titled "Methods of Measuring Growth."

43. Refer to chapter 5 in the textbook for a discussion in the section titled "Measurement of Cell Number."

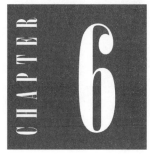

CHAPTER 6

Answer Key

1. a; d	**11.** b	**21.** d
2. b	**12.** c	**22.** e
3. c	**13.** b	**23.** f
4. a	**14.** a	**24.** c
5. a; d	**15.** b	**25.** a
6. d	**16.** c	**26.** b
7. b	**17.** b	**27.** d
8. b	**18.** b	**28.** a
9. d	**19.** a	**29.** b
10. b	**20.** a	**30.** d

31. ATP is 1) the major source of energy for endergonic reactions; 2) large amounts of energy released in chemical reactions is conserved by the formation of a high-energy phosphate bond on ADP, which makes ATP.

32. b

33. e

34. a

35. d

36. c

37. Oxygen in aerobic respiration; carbon dioxide, nitrate ion, and sulfate ion serve as final electron acceptors in anaerobic respiration.

38. Substrate phosphorylation

39. Oxidative phosphorylation

40. Photophosphorylation

41. End products may act as inhibitors of an allosteric enzyme in the pathway that leads to the end product. The change in an active site by the binding of an end product to the allosteric site may increase the binding to a substrate, and thus modulate the action of the enzyme.

42. Certain enzymes in eucaryotic cells are controlled by this process. The addition of a chemical group to an enzyme by covalent bonding may either increase or inhibit its catalytic action.

43. The presence of the substrate for the controlled enzymes induces the synthesis of the enzymes.

44. Glucose is a global repressor for many inducible enzymes because its catabolism reduces the concentration of cAMP, a molecule that is important for the induction of enzymes.

45. Two

46. ATP$\rightarrow$ADP + Pi

48. ATP$\rightarrow$ADP + Pi

52. ADP$\rightarrow$ATP; this is multiplied by two because two molecules of substrate are involved per glucose molecule.

55. ADP$\rightarrow$ATP; this is multiplied by two because two molecules of substrate are involved per glucose molecule.

56. Over reaction arrow numbered 52, write NAD + H+$\rightarrow$NADH; this is multiplied by two because two molecules of Glyceraldehyde 3-phosphate are converted to 1,3-Diphosphoglycerate.

57. An organic molecule acts as the final electron and hydrogen acceptor in fermentation to oxidize NADH.

58. The hydrogens and electrons of NADH are transferred to the electron transport chain, and NAD is generated.

For the additional practice section, the answer is found on Figure 6-14 and the corresponding text in chapter 6 of the textbook.

CHAPTER 7

Answer Key

1. c
2. d
3. d
4. b
5. a
6. e
7. a
8. c
9. b
10. d
11. a
12. a
13. b
14. e
15. b
16. c
17. c
18. e
19. a
20. b

21. DNA
22. Protein
23. Nuclear area in cytoplasm
24. Nuclear area in cytoplasm
25. Nucleus
26. At ribosome on endoplasmic reticulum
27. ACGU
28. None
29. Deoxyribonucleotide
30. Amino acid

For questions 31-33, refer to the textbook for a discussion of topics.

34. Repressor protein
35. P = promoter
36. O = operator
37. A = a structural gene for an enzyme
38. Enzyme production at the operon is blocked.
39. Enzyme production at the operon is induced.

Crossword Puzzle Answers:

Down:
1. rRNA
2. Conjugation
3. His
4. Transposon
5. mRNA
7. tRNA
8. Phenotype
9. Plasmid
12. PCR

Across:
4. Transformation
6. Genotype
10. Nucleotide
11. Mutation
12. Probe
13. DNA
14. Transduction

Answer Key

CHAPTER 8

Division names can be in any order for answers 1–8:

1. Gracilicutes
2. Gram-negative type cell wall; no spores; phototrophs; chemoautotrophs; chemoheterotrophs
3. Firmicutes
4. Gram-positive type cell wall; some may produce endospores; chemoheterotrophs
5. Tenericutes
6. No cell wall; no endospores; chemoheterotrophs with specific nutrient requirements
7. Mendosicutes
8. All archaea; no peptidoglycan in the cell wall; no fatty acids in lipids; rRNA base sequence is unique
9. b
10. a
11. b
12. a
13. Binomial nomenclature
14. First
15. Capitalized
16. Second
17. Lowercase
18. Italic
19. Underlining
20. Strain
21-22. Presence or absence of a cell wall; chemical composition of the cell wall
23. Organisms A and C may be related organisms. B is not likely to be related to A or C. DNA hybridization and other genetic tests may help to decide the relatedness of A and C.

24. b
25. h
26. d
27. i
28. a
29. c
30. f
31. e
32. g
33. j
34. a) Cell walls of archaea do not contain peptidoglycan; most bacterial walls do contain peptidoglycan; eucaryotes do not contain peptidoglycan in their cell walls; b) lipids of archaea do not contain fatty acids, as do bacteria and eucaryotes; c) the base sequence of archaeal rRNA is unique; d) Archaea survive in extreme environments.
35. Bacteria live in many different environments. Some procaryotes are unusual, and they have not been grown successfully in the laboratory. Mutations occur suddenly and randomly by a variety of gene transfer mechanisms, and by other means. Very few species are known to exhibit sexual mating. Not all bacteria have been discovered.
36. e
37. c
38. b
39. a
40. d

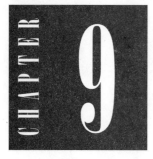

CHAPTER 9

Answer Key

1. e	**8.** f, j	**15.** e	**30.** a	**38.** b
2. h	**9.** d	**16.** c	**31.** b	**39.** c
3. g	**10.** a	**17.** e	**32.** a	**40.** a
4. a	**11.** a; b; c	**18.** b	**33.** c	**41.** c
5. i	**12.** d	**19.** a	**34.** b	**42.** b
6. b, c	**13.** b	**20.** c	**35.** d	**43.** d
7. j	**14.** d		**36.** d	**44.** a
			37. a; b; c	**45.** b

21-23. Answers may be in any order:
1) chemical nature of cell wall,
2) types of photosynthetic pigment molecules, and 3) types of reserve storage molecules

24. Pseudopodia

25. Mastigophora

26. Longitudinal fission

27. Adults are nonmotile; flagella are present in immature forms and gametes.

28. Cilia

29. Transverse fission; conjugation

46. Trophozoite is the active feeding stage of a protozoan; the cyst is the dormant, nonfeeding, thick-walled resistant stage.

47. A possible explanation may be that the larger size of the colonial form offers protection against some predators.

CHAPTER 10 Answer Key

1. d   **5.** h   **9.** a
2. f   **6.** i   **10.** b
3. c   **7.** j
4. g   **8.** e

11. Type of nucleic acid molecule, either DNA or RNA, and viruses are further divided by the number of strands of their nucleic acid.

12. d   **14.** e   **16.** a
13. c   **15.** f   **17.** b

18-20. icosahedral; helical; complex

21-26. See the section titled "Replication of Viruses," which describes the stages from attachment of a virus to a host cell, to the release of many virions after replication.

Replication Diagram: See Figure 10-6 in the textbook for assistance in labeling the virus-cell diagrams.

27. The lytic cycle produces a large number of virus particles immediately after the virus infection begins. Lysogeny occurs when viral DNA integrates into the host DNA and remains there for many generations of cell division. The lysogenic virus forms a prophage that does not harm the host cell until the lytic cycle of virus replication is induced. For your own practice, compare this to the concept of latency in animal viruses.

28. A prophage carries genetic properties, which, if transcribed by the host cell, will convert the host to one or more new capabilities. In some cases, this results in toxin production.

29. 1) Embryonated egg inoculations with virus; 2) cell cultures of various animal or plant tissues cultivated in tubes and bottles; 3) live animal inoculations

30. CPE refers to any number of distinct changes in the cells of a cell culture when a virus is infecting the culture. These changes are used to monitor virus presence and replication.

31. ID_{50} identifies the highest dilution that contains a virus capable of CPE. This technique measures the strength of virus numbers by identifying how many dilutions it takes before no CPE is seen.

32. The enzyme produces a DNA copy of the retroviral RNA molecule. The viral DNA is incorporated into the host cell chromosome.

Virus Model Exercise: If you want to experience holding an icosahedron, a 20-sided polyhedron, do this exercise. Many viruses have capsids with icosahedral symmetry.

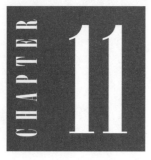

Answer Key

1. a; b (but that's not a fair answer)
2. d
3. d
4. b
5. c
6-8. See chapter 11 in the textbook to check your answers.
9. b
10. b
11. c
12. a
13. b
14. c
15. Descriptive, analytical, and experimental. See chapter 12 to check your descriptions of these types of investigations.
16. c
17. a
18. b
19. 0.003 percent
20. 0.0076 percent
21. 0.021 percent
22-23. See chapter 11 in the textbook to check your answers.
24. a
25. b
26. c
27. b
28. b
29. a
30. a

31. a
32. CDC guidelines for protecting patients and health care workers from the hazards of blood and body fluids; see Tables 11-5 and 11-6.
33. Any invasive medical procedure can facilitate entry of microorganisms. Can you identify one or more invasive medical procedures? Ask your instructor to check your answer.
34. The hospital is able to control incidence rates of nosocomial disease if this information is available.
35. Physicians in states F and G may especially be alerted to the possibility that penicillin may not treat *S. pneumoniae* infections successfully. Antimicrobial susceptibility testing is recommended for *S. pneumoniae* infections (see chapter 22). For those who want to know the states represented on this graph: A) Maryland; B) California; C) Oregon; D) Connecticut; E) Minnesota; F) Georgia; G) Tennessee.

CHAPTER 12 Answer Key

1-3. Answers may be given in any order: virulence, quantity of microbial invaders or toxins, and host resistance. See chapter 12 to check your descriptions.

4. c	**9.** b	**14.** a
5. b	**10.** b	**15.** c
6. d	**11.** a	**16.** b
7. a	**12.** a	**17.** b
8. b	**13.** b	

18. Lipopolysaccharide, especially lipid A component. See Figure 12-4 in the textbook.

19. Iron stress

20. Microorganisms mutate in response to gene transfer mechanisms. The expression of pathogenicity islands depends on environmental factors.

21. The closely-packed endothelial cells of cerebral capillaries, and a substantial basement membrane and astrocytes, form a barrier between blood capillaries and the central nervous system.

22. Some microorganisms exit capillaries at the dorsal root ganglia and enter the central nervous system. A few viruses travel across the barrier, especially in children whose basement membrane is not fully developed.

23. d	**25.** b	**27.** c
24. e	**26.** a	

Crossword Puzzle Answers:

Across:	Down:
1. Symptom	**2.** Pathogen
5. Hemolysis	**3.** Sign
8. LD	**4.** Hyaluronidase
10. Exofolin	**6.** Enzyme
11. Proteins	**7.** ID
12. Pleura	**9.** AIDS
14. Virulence	**11.** PCP
	13. CDC

CHAPTER 13 Answer Key

1. a	**10.** d	**19.** e
2. b	**11.** c	**20.** f
3. a	**12.** b	**21.** c
4. a	**13.** b	**22.** g
5. b	**14.** d	**23.** f
6. a	**15.** b	**24.** e
7. b	**16.** d	**25.** b
8. b	**17.** c	**26.** d
9. d	**18.** a	**27.** f

28. This is also known as antibody-mediated immunity. Humoral refers to circulating body fluids (humors) that contain immunoglobulin molecules produced by specific plasma cells from selected B cell clones.

29. This is also known as cell-mediated immunity. When activated by antigen, T lymphocytes send out cytokines to attract and activate macrophages, B cells, and other cells to the invasion site. T cells secrete cytokines to slow migration of macrophages away from the invasion site.

30. IgG	**36.** IgA
31. IgG, IgM, IgA	**37.** IgG
32. IgG, IgE, IgD	**38.** IgE
33. IgA	**39.** IgM
34. 2	**40.** IgG, IgM
35. 10	**41.** IgG

42. Refer to chapter 13 of the textbook and Figure 13-19 to compose your answer. Both IgM and IgG are produced in primary and secondary immune responses to the same antigen. IgM is always produced early but it persists for a short time. IgG is produced after IgM but it persists longer. Memory B and T cells allow for very rapid IgG production in higher concentration than in the primary response.

43. Primary challenge means the first exposure to an etiologic agent or vaccine. Secondary challenge means the second, or further, exposure to the same agent. IgM concentrations rise first and persist for weeks. IgG molecules rise in concentration after IgM molecules, but persist for months and years.

44. Memory B and T cells are partially activated by the primary challenge; they become fully active when challenged by the same antigen to which they react.

45. Vaccines act as antigens to stimulate the primary immune response without producing active disease. Memory cells are produced.

46. The secondary challenge refers to additional doses of a vaccine used to stimulate a stronger immune response.

47. g	**50.** h	**53.** d
48. i	**51.** c	**54.** b
49. a	**52.** e	**55.** f

56. See chapter 13, Figure 13-16 in the textbook to compare your answers.

CHAPTER **14** Answer Key

For checking your answers to 1-4, see chapter 14.

5. Types I, II, III

6. Immediate

7. Type IV

8. Delayed

For checking your answers to 9-10, see Chapter 14.

11. a	**24.** f	**37.** b
12. b	**25.** e	**38.** c
13. b	**26.** e	**39.** d
14. c	**27.** g	**40.** i
15. c	**28.** a	**41.** c
16. d	**29.** d	**42.** d
17. a	**30.** a	**43.** g
18. b	**31.** b	**44.** b
19. e	**32.** d	**45.** f
20. c	**33.** a	**46.** h
21. a	**34.** c	**47.** e
22. e	**35.** b	**48.** a
23. d	**36.** d	

49. The incidence of childhood diseases has declined dramatically during the 20th century in those developed countries with childhood vaccination programs. When children are vaccinated against early childhood diseases before they enter daycare and school, families benefit by fewer illnesses, fewer absenses, and lower medical expenses. The public health generally improves as the majority a community are vaccinated against the most common disease agents. This means that the herd immunity is increased to these diseases, so etiologic agents have less opportunity to establish disease in susceptible individuals in the community.

CHAPTER 15 Answer Key

1. b	**5.** e	**9.** i	**13.** h
2. d	**6.** f	**10.** b	**14.** a
3. a	**7.** j	**11.** d	**15.** c
4. c	**8.** e	**12.** g	

16. Any opening in the skin allows the entrance of microorganisms.

17. Boil (furuncle): a pus-containing lesion

Carbuncle (abscess): open lesions develop when a boil spreads and produces deeper infections

Impetigo: blisters (vesicles) develop

Scalded-skin syndrome: the loss of the outermost epidermal cells caused by the bacterial toxin

Toxic shock syndrome: a multisystem disease with a rash induced by toxin

18. Magnesium bound by the tampon fibers promotes toxin production by native *S. aureus.*

19. Tineas, candidiasis, subcutaneous mycoses including sporotrichosis, chromomycoses, and mycetomas. Most are transmitted by direct contact with an infected individual or animal, or indirectly by contact with a fomite.

20. The viruses establish latency, a dormant period in the virus cycle that occurs in host cells; the virus can activate under certain conditions causing virulent disease.

21. Measles, rubella, herpes simplex infections, varicella-zoster infections, roseola infantum, warts, erythema infectiosum.

22. The bacteria are capable of growing in environments with very minimal nutrients such as containers of water, liquid soaps, and weak disinfectants.

23. The patient must move or be moved frequently.

24. The developing fetus is infected by the virus which produces severe defects in fetal development.

25. Heart disease, mental retardation, deafness, blindness

26. c
27. c
28. e
29. a
30. c
31. b
32. c
33. b
34. b
35. c
36. a
37. a

CHAPTER 16 Answer Key

1. c
2. i
3. j
4. l
5. r

6. g
7. o
8. t
9. h
10. a

11. f
12. e
13. b
14. p
15. s

16. q
17. d
18. m
19. n
20. k

21. The letter B is placed at b, c, g, i, j, l, m, n, o, p, q, r.
22. The letter F is placed at a, d, f, k.
23. Nose, paranasal sinuses, middle ear, pharynx, tonsils
24. Trachea, bronchi, alveolar spaces, interstitial tissues of lung
25. a
26. Immunizations in early childhood
27. Many staphyloccal strains exhibit resistance to penicillins.
28. Many strains of *H. influenzae* exhibit resistance to multiple drugs at once.
29. Mycoplasmas and chlamydias have no cell walls so they are not susceptible to penicillin drugs.

30. Histoplasmosis, coccidioidomycosis, blastomycosis

31. c
32. b
33. a
34. d
35. d

36. a
37. d
38. b
39. c
40. e

41. c
42. e
43. b
44. a
45. b

46. a
47. b
48. a
49. a

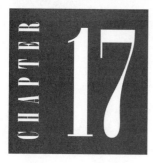

CHAPTER 17

Answer Key

1. Oral genera: *Streptococcus, Lactobacillus, Actinomyces, Candida albicans, Entamoeba gingivalis.* Oropharynx genera: *Moraxella, Bacteroides, Veillonella.*

2. Small intestine: yeast, *Candida albicans.* Colon: Gram-positive bacteria: *Bacteroides, Fusobacterium, Clostridium perfringens, Peptostreptococcus, Peptococcus.* Yeast, *Candida albicans.* Gram-negative bacteria: *Escherichia coli, Klebsiella, Proteus, Enterobacter, Pseudomonas.*

3. Liver: HAV, HBV, HCV. Intestine: Rotavirus, Norwalk virus, Coxsackievirus, Echovirus, Enterovirus, CMV.

4. The microorganisms trapped in food particles escape the action of gastric secretions.

5. c   8. b   11. c   14. b
6. b   9. c   12. b   15. b
7. a   10. b   13. b

16. The disease symptoms are primarily caused by the neurotoxin contained in infected food.

17. A large population of a pathogenic organism and its metabolic products including toxins growing in the intestine are responsible for disease.

18. The presence of toxins in food is responsible for disease.

19. Drink bottled water and brush teeth with bottled water, or boil and filter local water before drinking. Adequately treat water with chlorine or iodine solutions. Avoid fresh fruit and vegetables washed in local water. Do not use ice made from local untreated water.

20. *Yersinia enterocolitica*

21. *Clostridium difficile*

22. *Entamoeba histolytica*

23. *Campylobacter jejuni*

24. Cytomegalovirus

25. *Shigella sonnei*

26. Mumps virus

27. *Vibrio parahaemolyticus*

28. Hepatitis viruses: HAV, HBV, HCV

29. *Clostridium botulinum*

30. *Vibrio cholerae*

31. *Salmonella typhi*

32. *Giardia lamblia*

33. *Escherichia coli*, enterotoxin producer

34. *Escherichia coli* 0157:H7, shiga-like toxin producer

35. b   37. c   39. a
36. a   38. b   40. c

41. Liver; fecal-oral route

42. Parotid gland; Oral or respiratory secretions

43. Any organ, commonly GI tract; transplacental, kissing, sexual intercourse, blood transfusions, organ transplants, fomites

Crossword Puzzle Answers:

Across:
  1. Gum
  5. Strepto
  7. Itis
  9. Sucrose
  12. Cementum
  13. Periodontal
  14. Oral

Down:
  2. Mutans
  3. Floss
  4. Caries
  6. Plaque
  8. Inflamed
  10. Enamel
  11. Actino

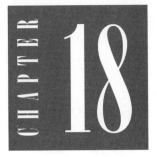

CHAPTER 18

Answer Key

1. The urethra in females is shorter, allowing microorganisms from external surfaces to ascend into the bladder faster. Infrequent urination allows colonization of urethra and bladder. Microbes may ascend in the ureters to produce kidney infection.

2. Nongonococcal urethritis: *Chlamydia trachomatis, Mycoplasma genitalium, M. hominis, Ureaplasma urealyticum.* UTI: *E. coli* or other gram-negative bacteria of intestinal origin.

3. *Chlamydia trachomatis, Neisseria gonorrhoeae, Bacteroides fragilis*

4. Yeast: *Candida albicans.* Protozoa: *Trichomonas vaginalis*

5. An exogenous infection is caused by an organism not usually found on/in the body.

6. An endogenous infection is caused by an organism or virus found on/in the body.

7. The initial infection and re-infections are exogenous. The virus establishes latency, a dormant phase inside nervous tissue, and erupts into endogenous disease under certain conditions.

8. f	**15.** e	**22.** a	**29.** a, c
9. d	**16.** b	**23.** c	**30.** d
10. b	**17.** c	**24.** c	**31.** d
11. e	**18.** a	**25.** a	**32.** c
12. c	**19.** c	**26.** e	
13. a	**20.** c	**27.** a	
14. c	**21.** b	**28.** d	

33. See the textbook, chapter 18 to check your answer.

34. Both chlamydias and mycoplasmas are responsible for nongonococcal urethritis. Chlamydias cause genital infections, PID, conjunctivitis of newborn delivered from an infected mother, and some types cause LGV.

35. *Haemophilus ducreyi*

36. *Calymmatobacterium granulomatis*

37. *Chlamydia trachomatis*

38. *Trichomonas vaginalis*

39. *Treponema pallidum*

40. Herpes simplex type 2, sometimes type 1

41. Human immunodeficiency virus

42. *Chlamydia trachomatis* plus others, see answer to #34

43. *Candida albicans*

44. *Gardnerella vaginalis,* and some anaerobes

45. *C. trachomatis, N. gonorrhoeae, B. fragilis*

46. *Leptospira interrogans* type *icterohaemorrhagiae*

47. Papillomaviruses

48. c	**50.** c	**52.** d
49. b	**51.** d	

CHAPTER 19

Answer Key

1. The central and peripheral nervous systems are sterile. In severe septicemia, microorganisms may migrate into the brain and spinal fluid from the blood. Microorganisms and their toxins may enter neural tissue by the eustachian tube, mastoid process, peripheral nerves, cribriform plate, and trauma.

2. *Neisseria meningitidis, Haemophilus influenzae, Streptococcus pneumoniae, Listeria monocytogenes*

3. See textbook, chapter 19 to check your answers.

4. *Cryptococcus neoformans,* and species of *Absidia, Mucor, Rhizopus, Mortierella*

5. *Naegleria fowleri, Acanthamoeba, Toxoplasma gondii, Trypanosoma brucei gambiense or T. b. rhodesiense*

6. See textbook to check your answer.

7. Prions are heat-resistant protein particles, with a latency period of months or years. Viruses are composed of nucleic acid molecules bounded by a protein capsid and perhaps other structures; infections are acute and some viruses may establish a latent infection.

8. Microorganisms, antibiotics, and some antibodies have difficulty crossing the bloodstream into the brain and meninges because of the selective permeability of the capillaries.

9. Eye: trauma, bloodstream, infected implants. Ear: penetrating wound, bloodstream, eustachian tube.

10. b	13. h	16. g, j	19. f
11. b,c	14. d	17. k	20. a
12. e	15. i	18. a	21. b,c

22. *Naegleria fowleri, Acanthamoeba*

23. Staphylococci

24. WEE virus

25. *Neisseria meningitidis*

26. *Chlamydia trachomatis*

27. Poliovirus

28. *Haemophilus aegyptius*

29. Rabies virus

30. *Clostridium tetani*

31. *Trypanosoma brucei gambiense* and *T. b. rhodesiense*

32. Prion

33. Herpes simplex 1 or others

34. Acute mastoiditis, meningitis, brain abscess, hearing impairment

35. Salk (killed injectable) and Sabin (oral, live attenuated) vaccines

36. Immunocompromised status of patient, trauma, paranasal sinus infections

37. Tetanus toxoid injections

38. d	40. b	42. d
39. e	41. d	

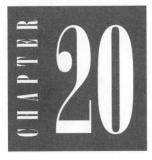

CHAPTER **20**

Answer Key

1. Circulating cells include red blood cells for oxygen and carbon dioxide gas exchanges; macrophages, white blood cells, and platelets for immune defense. Sessile cells are macrophages located in the organs for immune defense. These include the Kupffer cells of the liver, osteoclasts of bone, and microglial cells of nerve tissue, and others.

2. a	**5.** a	**8.** b	**11.** b
3. b	**6.** b	**9.** a	**12.** b
4. b	**7.** a	**10.** b	**13.** b

14-25. See Table 20-2 in the textbook to check your answers.

26. The mosquito larvae develop in stagnant pools and swamps. These must be drained or sprayed with insecticide or some other means of mosquito control. Any small pool of water in the backyard breeds mosquitoes. They are resistant to insecticide sprays. There is no vaccine available yet. Infected wild and domestic animals and infected humans are reservoirs.

27. Yellow fever
28. Plague
29. Rocky Mountain spotted fever
30. Relapsing fever
31. Malaria
32. American trypanosomiasis
33. Leishmaniasis
34. Lyme disease
35. Relapsing fever

36. *Brucella abortus* or others
37. *Leishmania donovani*
38. *Franciscella tularensis*
39. *Yersinia pestis*
40. *Borrelia recurrentis*
41. *Borrelia burgdorferi*
42. Epstein-Barr virus
43. *Plasmodium vivax* and others
44. *Leishmania braziliensis*
45. *Rickettsia rickettsii*

46. Wear long-sleeved shirts and long pants, use insect repellant sprays on clothes and skin, and place fine netting around bed to keep mosquitoes from biting at night.

47. Ecological relationships of parasite, vector, reservoir, and hosts to a specific niche serve to limit the distribution of some diseases.

48. See textbook to check your answers.

49. b	**51.** b	**53.** e
50. a	**52.** c	

CHAPTER 21 Answer Key

1-4. See Table 21-1 to compare your answer.

   5. See chapter 21 to compare your answer.

   6. a

   7. a

   8. a

   9. b

 10. b

 11. a

 12. a

 13. a

 14. b

 15. a

 16. b

 17. a

 18. b

 19. a

 20. a

21. To sterilize the metal so it does not contain organisms to contaminate a culture; before inoculating a culture medium and after inoculation to avoid contamination of the laboratory or workers.

22. See chapter 21 to compare your answer.

23. a

24. a

25. b

26. b

27. a

28. a

29. c

30. c

31. An enzyme activated by visible light called photoreactivating enzyme (PRE) repairs UV damage of DNA. The enzyme breaks the thymine dimer bond so normal base pairing of thymine to the opposite adenine is established.

32. Cells exposed to UV irradiation and then placed in a dark and cold environment for an extended period of time may have the UV damage repaired by dark repair enzymes. These enzymes excise the thymine dimers and replace them with thymine nucleotides so normal base-pairing to the opposite adenine bases is established.

33. The chemical changes induced by visible light exposure in an oxygen environment.

34. a

35. a

36. d

37. c

38. c

39. a

40. b

41. b

42. b

43. b

44. a

45. a

46. b

47. b

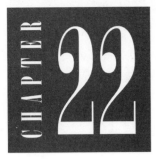

CHAPTER 22

Answer Key

1. c
2. a
3. d
4. e
5. b
6. a
7. b
8. c
9. c
10. c
11. e
12. a
13. d
14. e
15. b
16. c
17. a
18. c
19. d
20. d

21. The β-lactamases are produced by microorganisms that are resistant to some antibiotics in the penicillin and cephalosporin families of drugs. The testing for β-lactamase activity for the etiological agent of a patient's infection is essential to selecting the appropriate antimicrobial therapy.

22. The therapeutic dose for *S. aureus* is not provided by the concentration of ampicillin in the disk.

23. The interpretation of results must be based on pure cultures. Contaminating organisms may have a different response to antimicrobials than does the etiological agent.

24. The therapeutic dose for each species is different.

25. Measurement in millimeters of the clear zone showing no growth around the paper disk that contains an antimicrobial agent. These mm values are compared to a standard interpretative chart to determine R, S, and I results.

26. c
27. a
28. b
29. c
30. a
31. c
32. b
33. a
34. c
35. b
36. a
37. d
38. a
39. e
40. b

41 and 42. See chapter 22 to compare your answers.

CHAPTER 23 Answer Key

1. e

2. g

3. b

4. a

5. g

6. d

7. a

8. f

9. e

10. b

11-13. See chapter 23 to compare your answer.

14. b

15. a

16. c

17. b

18. b

19. b and c

20. a

21. See chapter 23 to compare your answer.

22. Sunlight energy is required by photosynthetic producers, and it is strongest at the surface of water.

23. See chapter 23 to compare your answer.

24. Hydrothermal vents have increased pressure; higher temperature; no light; with animal life dependent on chemosynthetic bacterial producers near hydrothermal vents. Other marine environments are colder, with less pressure near the surface where aquatic photosynthetic producers live.

25. b; h

26. a; b

27. c; f

28. h

29. a; b

30. g

31. a

32. f or h

33. h

34. b

35. d

36. c

37. h

38. f

39. d

40. a

41. a

42. c

43. b

44. b

45. a

46. d

47. b

48. c

49. c

50. e

51. d

52. b

53. d

54. d

55. See chapter 23 to compare your answer.

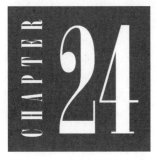

Answer Key

1. e
2. b
3. k
4. d
5. i
6. n
7. f
8. a
9. g
10. l
11. e
12. c
13. j
14. e
15. h
16. h
17. n
18. b
19. q
20. a
21. Heating methods coagulate proteins and reduce water activity, which stops microbial action. Cold slows, but does not stop, enzyme activity of cells in food.
22 and **23.** Ethyl alcohol and carbon dioxide
24. Yeast, *Saccharomyces cerevisiae*
25. Ethyl alcohol
26. *Acetobacter aceti,* and other acetic acid producing bacteria,
27. Acetic acid
28. b
29. a

30. c
31. i
32. d
33. d; f; g
34. e
35. c
36. a; i
37. j
38. k
39. j
40. h
41. B for 28, 29, 30, 31, 32, 34, 35, 36, and 38
42. Y for 33 and 40
43. M for 37 and 39
44. LA for 28, 29, 30, 31, 34, 35, 36
45. *Saccharomyces cerevisiae*
46. *Acetobacter aceti*
47. *Streptococcus diacetylactis*
48. Fecal contamination has occurred.
49. In water and milk, coliform bacteria indicate contamination by fecal material and perhaps pathogenic organisms.
50. See chapter 24 to compare your answer.
51. c
52. a
53. c
54. a
55. a
56. a